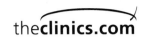

MEDICAL CLINICS
OF NORTH AMERICA

Integrated Care for the
Complex Medically Ill

GUEST EDITORS
Frits J. Huyse, MD, PhD
Friedrich C. Stiefel, MD, PhD

July 2006 • Volume 90 • Number 4

SAUNDERS

An Imprint of Elsevier, Inc.
PHILADELPHIA LONDON TORONTO MONTREAL SYDNEY TOKYO

W.B. SAUNDERS COMPANY
A Division of Elsevier Inc.

1600 John F. Kennedy Boulevard • Suite 1800 • Philadelphia, Pennsylvania 19103-2899

http://www.theclinics.com

MEDICAL CLINICS OF NORTH AMERICA Volume 90, Number 4
July 2006 ISSN 0025-7125
Editor: Rachel Glover ISBN 1-4160-3888-4

Medical Clinics of North America (ISSN 0025-7125) is published bimonthly by W.B. Saunders, 360 Park Avenue South, New York, NY 10010-1710. Business and editorial offices: 1600 John F. Kennedy Boulevard, Suite 1800, Philadelphia, PA 19103-2899. Accounting and circulation offices: 6277 Sea Harbor Drive, Orlando, FL 32887-4800. Periodicals postage paid at New York, NY, and additional mailing offices. Subscription prices are USD 145 per year for US individuals, USD 260 per year for US institutions, USD 75 per year for US students, USD 185 per year for Canadian individuals, USD 330 per year for Canadian institutions, USD 210 per year for international individuals, USD 330 per year for international institutions and USD 110 per year for Canadian and foreign students/residents. To receive student/resident rate, orders must be accompanied by name of affiliated institution, date of term, and the *signature* of program/residency coordinator on institution letterhead. Orders will be billed at individual rate until proof of status is received. Foreign air speed delivery is included in all *Clinics* subscription prices. All prices are subject to change without notice. POSTMASTER: Send address changes to *Medical Clinics of North America,* Elsevier Periodicals Customer Service, 6277 Sea Harbor Drive, Orlando, FL 32887-4800. **Customer Service: 1-800-654-2452 (US). From outside of the USA, call (+1) 407-345-1000. E-mail: hhspcs@harcourt.com.**

Reprints. For copies of 100 or more, of articles in this publication, please contact the Commercial Reprints Department, Elsevier Inc., 360 Park Avenue South, New York, New York 10010-1710. Tel.: (+1) (212) 633-3813; Fax: (+1) (212) 462-1935; E-mail: reprints@elsevier.com.

Medical Clinics of North America is also published in Spanish by McGraw-Hill Interamericana Editores S. A., P.O. Box 5-237, 06500 Mexico, D.F., Mexico.

Medical Clinics of North America is covered in *Index Medicus, Current Contents, ASCA, Excerpta Medica, Science Citation Index,* and *ISI/BIOMED.*

Printed in the United States of America.

GOAL STATEMENT

The goal of *Medical Clinics of North America* is to keep practicing physicians up to date with current clinical practice by providing timely articles reviewing the state of the art in patient care.

ACCREDITATION

The *Medical Clinics of North America* is planned and implemented in accordance with the Essential Areas and Policies of the Accreditation Council for Continuing Medical Education (ACCME) through the joint sponsorship of the University of Virginia School of Medicine and Elsevier. The University of Virginia School of Medicine is accredited by the ACCME to provide continuing medical education for physicians.

The University of Virginia School of Medicine designates this educational activity for a maximum of 90 *AMA PRA Category 1 Credits*™. Physicians should only claim credit commensurate with the extent of their participation in the activity.

The American Medical Association has determined that physicians not licensed in the US who participate in this CME activity are eligible for *AMA PRA Category 1 Credits*™.

Category 1 credit can be earned by reading the text material, taking the CME examination online at *http://www.theclinics.com/home/cme*, and completing the evaluation. After taking the test, you will be required to review any and all incorrect answers. Following completion of the test and evaluation, your credit will be awarded and you may print your certificate.

FACULTY DISCLOSURE/CONFLICT OF INTEREST

The University of Virginia School of Medicine, as an ACCME accredited provider, endorses and strives to comply with the Accreditation Council for Continuing Medical Education (ACCME) Standards of Commercial Support, Commonwealth of Virginia statutes, University of Virginia policies and procedures, and associated federal and private regulations and guidelines on the need for disclosure and monitoring of proprietary and financial interests that may affect the scientific integrity and balance of content delivered in continuing medical education activities under our auspices.

The University of Virginia School of Medicine requires that all CME activities accredited through this institution be developed independently and be scientifically rigorous, balanced and objective in the presentation/discussion of its content, theories and practices.

All authors/editors participating in an accredited CME activity are expected to disclose to the readers relevant financial relationships with commercial entities occurring within the past 12 months (such as grants or research support, employee, consultant, stock holder, member of speakers bureau, etc.). The University of Virginia School of Medicine will employ appropriate mechanisms to resolve potential conflicts of interest to maintain the standards of fair and balanced education to the reader. Questions about specific strategies can be directed to the Office of Continuing Medical Education, University of Virginia School of Medicine, Charlottesville, Virginia.

The authors/editors listed below have identified no professional or financial affiliations for themselves or their spouse/partner:
David Clarke, MBBS, PhD, FRANZCP; Peter de Jonge, PhD; Leonard E. Egede, MD, MS; Rijk O.B. Gans, MD, PhD; Rachel Glover, Acquisitions Editor; Frits J. Huyse, MD, PhD; Corine H.M. Latour, CNS, RN; Antonio Lobo, MD, PhD; John S. Lyons, PhD; Johan Ormel, PhD; Judith G. M. Rosmalen, PhD, MA; Stephen M. Saravay, MD; Joris P. J. Slaets, MD, PhD; Graeme Smith, MD, BS, DPM, FRANZCP; Wolfgang Söllner, MD; Friedrich C. Stiefel, MD, PhD; Nynke van der Wal, ANP; and, Lawson R. Wulsin, MD.

The authors/editors listed below identified the following professional or financial affiliations for themselves or their spouse/partner:
Roger Kathol, MD, is employed by, is a consultant for, and has stock/ownership in, Cartesian Solutions, Inc.
Kurt Kroenke, MD, is an independent contractor and a consultant for Eli Lilly and Wyeth Pharmaceuticals, an independent contractor for Pfizer, and is on the advisory committee/board for Eli Lilly.
Harold A. Pincus, MD, is employed by University of Pittsburg Medical Center, Columbia University, and New York Presbyterian Hospital, is a consultant for Cisco Systems, and is on the speaker's bureau for Comprehensive Neurosciences.

Disclosure of Discussion of non-FDA approved uses for pharmaceutical products and/or medical devices:
The University of Virginia School of Medicine, as an ACCME provider, requires that all faculty presenters identify and disclose any "off label" uses for pharmaceutical and medical device products. The University of Virginia School of Medicine recommends that each physician fully review all the available data on new products or procedures prior to instituting them with patients.

TO ENROLL

To enroll in the Medical Clinics of North America Continuing Medical Education program, call customer service at 1-800-654-2452 or visit us online at *http://www.theclinics.com/home/cme*. The CME program is available to subscribers for an additional fee of USD 205.

FORTHCOMING ISSUES

RECENT ISSUES

GUEST EDITORS

FRITS J. HUYSE, MD, PhD, Associate Professor of Consultation/Liaison Psychiatry, Department of General Internal Medicine, University Medical Center Groningen, Groningen, The Netherlands

FRIEDRICH C. STIEFEL, MD, PhD, Professor of Psychiatry, Service de Psychiatrie de Liaison, Centre Hospitalier Universitaire Vaudois, Lausanne, Switzerland

CONTRIBUTORS

DAVID CLARKE, MBBS, PhD, FRANZCP, Associate Professor, School of Psychology, Psychiatry and Psychological Medicine, Monash University, Clayton, Victoria, Australia

PETER DE JONGE, PhD, Assistant Professor, Departments of Internal Medicine and Psychiatry, University of Groningen, The Netherlands

BENJAMIN G. DRUSS, MD, MPH, Rosalynn Carter Chair in Mental Health, Emory University, Rollins School of Public Health, Atlanta, Georgia

LEONARD E. EGEDE, MD, MS, Associate Professor and Director, Center for Health Disparities Research, Division of General Internal Medicine, Medical University of South Carolina, Charleston, South Carolina; Director, Charleston VA Targeted Research Enhancement Program, Ralph H. Johnson VAMC, Charleston, South Carolina

RIJK O.B. GANS, MD, PhD, Professor of Medicine, University Medical Center Groningen, Groningen, The Netherlands

FRITS J. HUYSE, MD, PhD, Associate Professor of Consultation/Liaison Psychiatry, Department of General Internal Medicine, University Medical Center Groningen, Groningen, The Netherlands

ROGER KATHOL, MD, President, Cartesian Solutions, Inc., Burnsville, Minnesota; Adjunct Professor, Departments of Internal Medicine and Psychiatry, University of Minnesota, Minneapolis, Minnesota

KURT KROENKE, MD, Professor, Department of Medicine, Indiana University School of Medicine; Research Scientist, Regenstrief Institute, Indianapolis, Indiana

CORINE H.M. LATOUR, CNS, RN, Consultation-liaison Psychiatric Nurse, Psychiatric Consultation and Liaison Service, VU University Medical Center, Amsterdam, The Netherlands

ANTONIO LOBO, MD, PhD, Professor and Chair, Department of Psychiatry, Universidad de Zaragoza, Zaragoza, Spain

JOHN S. LYONS, PhD, Professor of Psychiatry and Community Medicine, Feinberg School of Medicine, Northwestern University, Chicago, Illinois

JOHAN ORMEL, PhD, Professor and Chair, Department of Social Psychiatry and Psychiatric Epidemiology, University Medical Center of Groningen, Groningen, The Netherlands

HAROLD ALAN PINCUS, MD, Vice Chair, Strategic Initiatives, Department of Psychiatry, Columbia University; Director of Quality and Outcomes Research, New York-Presbyterian Hospital; New York State Psychiatric Institute, New York, New York

JUDITH G.M. ROSMALEN, PhD, MA, Research Scientist, Department of Psychiatry, University Medical Center Groningen; Graduate School of Behavioral and Cognitive Neurosciences, University of Groningen, Groningen, The Netherlands; Graduate School for Experimental Psychopathology, The Netherlands

STEVEN M. SARAVAY, MD, Clinical Professor, Department of Psychiatry, Albert Einstein College of Medicine, New Hyde Park, New York

JORIS P.J. SLAETS, MD, PhD, Professor of Geriatrics, Department of Internal Medicine, University Medical Center Groningen, Groningen, The Netherlands

GRAEME SMITH, MD, BS, DPM, FRANZCP, Professor Emeritus, School of Psychology, Psychiatry and Psychological Medicine, Monash University, Clayton, Victoria, Australia

WOLFGANG SÖLLNER, MD, Associate Professor of Psychosomatics and Psychotherapy, General Hospital Nürnberg, Nürnberg, Germany

FRIEDRICH C. STIEFEL, MD, PhD, Professor of Psychiatry, Service de Psychiatrie de Liaison, Centre Hospitalier Universitaire Vaudois, Lausanne, Switzerland

NYNKE VAN DER WAL, ANP, Consultation-liaison Psychiatric Nurse, Consultant Integrated Care, Department of General Internal Medicine, University Medical Center Groningen, Groningen, The Netherlands

LAWSON R. WULSIN, MD, Professor of Psychiatry and Family Medicine, University of Cincinnati, Cincinnati, Ohio

CONTENTS

> It may appear self-evident that the integrated care of patients who
> have a complex or chronic illness is a necessity whose proper appli-
> cation will result in better health outcomes achieved as economically
> as possible. The uncritical application of integrated interventions
> produced disappointing results that prompted health care providers
> and theorists to revisit the underlying concepts and methodologies
> that were used. There is a realization that the complexity of the inter-
> vention and the target patients are such that existing methods of
> study need to be complemented by in-depth exploration using non-
> traditional methods, including qualitative ones. Recent develop-
> ments in theoretic constructs give promise of better answers to the
> question, "What works for whom in what context?".

> Concurrent general medical and psychiatric illnesses frequently oc-
> cur in the same individual, yet are assessed and treated in health
> care systems worldwide as though a relationship between the
> two did not exist. This article reviews evidence about the negative
> impact that segregated behavioral health and medical business
> practices, care management, and clinician intervention have on

clinical, functional, and financial outcomes. It discusses integrated care models that lead to health improvement and decrease the total cost of care. Finally, it delineates general steps that are needed to move from a fragmented to an integrated health system.

This article introduces the metabolic syndrome as a clinical pheno-type with consequences for diagnosis and treatment that go be-yond the different clinical specialties involved. A life-course approach is suggested as a means of understanding the complex interrelations between the metabolic syndrome, depression, and cardiovascular disease. Pathophysiologic mechanisms that these conditions share are discussed in detail. These considerations pro-vide arguments for a more integrative approach to patients in gen-eral that surpass the current disease-centered services such as endocrinology, psychiatry, and cardiology.

In scenarios that predict the future of health service delivery in the Western world, the rapid increase in frail elderly patients is seen as one of the major challenges of health care in addition to the care of the chronic medically ill. In this article the relation between age, frailty, comorbidity, and disability is elaborated further, a method to detect frail patients quickly is introduced, and its relation to complexity is explored. An argument for patient-tailored inte-grated care in frail elderly patients is made. At the same time, the argument will be made that standard evidence-based care can be delivered for patients who have a negative screen on frailty.

Half of all outpatient encounters are precipitated by physical com-plaints, of which one third to one half are medically unexplained symptoms, and 20% to 25% are chronic or recurrent. Many of the patients suffer from one or more discrete symptoms, whereas others have functional somatic syndromes. Individual symptoms and so-matic syndromes are associated with impaired quality of life, in-creased health care use, and diminished patient and provider satisfaction. This article provides an overview of (1) unexplained symptoms and somatization; (2) limitations of *Diagnostic and Statistical Manual of Mental Disorders, Fourth Edition* in classifying somatoform disorders; (3) predictors of psychiatric comorbidity in patients who have physical symptoms; and (4) measurement and management of symptoms.

Disease-Focused or Integrated Treatment: Diabetes and Depression
Leonard E. Egede

Diabetes and depression are chronic debilitating conditions that are associated with significant morbidity, mortality, and health care costs. Most patients who have diabetes are treated in primary care settings; however, multiple studies have shown that recognition and treatment of depression is less than optimal in this setting. This article reviews the literature on the adverse health outcomes of the coexistence of diabetes and depression, the challenges of treating coexisting diabetes and depression in a fragmented health care system, and the need for integrated care as a strategy to improve the quality of care for patients with complex medical illnesses (eg, patients who have coexisting diabetes and depression).

Models of Integrated Care
Lawson R. Wulsin, Wolfgang Söllner, and Harold Alan Pincus

This article describes the range of options for integrating medicine and psychiatry, with a focus on the advantages and limitations of each model. The models were developed in different countries with specific health care cultures. This article illustrates the range of in- and outpatient options as currently practiced, with case reports from practitioners when possible, and describes qualifications for practicing in each model, the settings, the patient populations, the relevant financial issues, and the advantages and disadvantages of practicing in each model. It closes with comments on the next steps for advancing integrated care and the barriers to be overcome.

Case and Care Complexity in the Medically Ill
Peter de Jonge, Frits J. Huyse, and Friedrich C. Stiefel

The concept of complexity is described increasingly in the medical literature and refers to the care needs of patients who have multi-morbid conditions and the organizational structure of health care systems. This article provides an overview of the literature on this concept and discusses the need to reconcile case and care complexity. Case complexity has been operationalized in several ways. Conversely, the operationalization of care complexity has drawn much less attention. As an example, an empiric model to describe the interrelations of several indicators of care complexity is presented.

The Complexity of Communication in an Environment with Multiple Disciplines and Professionals: Communimetrics and Decision Support

John S. Lyons

Accurate and efficient communication among all the parties is an important component of providing efficient and effective medical care to patients who have complex needs. The evolution of clinimetric measurement approaches designed to be congruent with the clinical process into communimetric tools designed to communicate the clinical process to wider audiences allows the use of technology to support improved care. Computerized medicine offers many opportunities for speeding up the communication of data and thereby improving the efficiency and effectiveness of medical care. The use of communimetric tools within this information environment represents an important opportunity to bridge the quality chasm.

Identifiers, or "Red Flags," of Complexity and Need for Integrated Care

Frits J. Huyse, Friedrich C. Stiefel, and Peter de Jonge

Because complex medical patients are a subgroup of the medical population and because complexity assessment involves extra effort, preselection of these patients through identifiers is necessary. There is no best identifier for complexity, and the one most suitable for the population served should be selected. This article provides a table with potential identifiers and discusses the difference between disease-oriented screening and treatment and a more generic approach such as complexity screening and complexity management.

Operationalizing Integrated Care on a Clinical Level: the INTERMED Project

Friedrich C. Stiefel, Frits J. Huyse, Wolfgang Söllner, Joris P.J. Slaets, John S. Lyons, Corine H.M. Latour, Nynke van der Wal, and Peter de Jonge

During the last 10 years the INTERMED method has been developed as a generic method for the assessment of bio-psychosocial health risks and health needs and for planning of integrated treatment. The INTERMED has been conceptualized to counteract divisions and fragmentation of medical care. Designed to enhance the communication between patients and the health providers as well as between different professions and disciplines, the INTERMED is a visualized, action-oriented decision-support tool. This article presents various aspects of the INTERMED, such as its relevance, description, scoring, the related patient interview and treatment planning, scientific evaluation, implementation, and support for the method.

ELSEVIER
SAUNDERS

Med Clin N Am 90 (2006) xiii–xiv

THE MEDICAL
CLINICS
OF NORTH AMERICA

Foreword

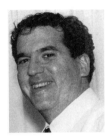

Benjamin G. Druss, MD, MPH

Comorbidity and complexity are increasingly the rule rather than the exception in clinical care. Society's success in treating acute illnesses has resulted in longer lives but also increasing prevalence, burden, and costs of chronic conditions. Chronicity, in turn, is associated invariably with high levels of comorbidity; however, clinical training, reimbursement, and research funding all remain organized around discrete clinical conditions. The result is a growing disconnect between the health system, which focuses on single diseases, and patients' clinical needs, which often span multiple providers, disciplines, and systems of care.

This important issue of the *Medical Clinics of North America*, edited by Frits Huyse and Friedrich Stiefel, seeks to understand how better to deliver care for the "complex medically ill," patients who have multiple medical, mental, psychosocial, or functional problems. Rather than focus on specific comorbidities, it addresses the broad themes regarding the identification, assessment, and management of these vulnerable patients. Many of the articles point toward integrated approaches as promising strategies for improving these patients' care.

The articles are written by many of the world's experts on these topics, and provide a combination of conceptual depth and empiric rigor. The international range of authors and study settings are a testament to how themes of complexity and comorbidity cut across multiple countries and settings of care.

The recently-released Institute of Medicine report "Improving the Quality of Health Care for Mental and Substance Use Conditions" found that

doi:10.1016/j.mcna.2006.05.007

deficits in quality of care for persons with behavioral conditions were as great or greater than the problems faced by persons with other medical problems. Many of these gaps result from fragmentation within the general and behavioral health system, and between the behavioral health and general medical systems. One of the most promising ways of understanding and improving care across these sectors is to understand and improve care for patients whose needs cut across them. This issue provides an invaluable step in that direction.

Benjamin G. Druss, MD, MPH
Emory University
Rollins School of Public Health
1518 Clifton Road, NE, Room 606
Atlanta, GA 30322, USA

E-mail address: bdruss@sph.emory.edu

THE MEDICAL
CLINICS
OF NORTH AMERICA

ELSEVIER
SAUNDERS

Med Clin N Am 90 (2006) xv–xviii

Preface

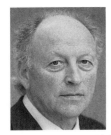 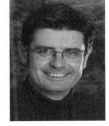

Frits J. Huyse, MD, PhD   Friedrich C. Stiefel, MD, PhD
Guest Editors

In the decades after the Second World War, the future of medicine seemed bright, almost without limits. Infectious diseases could be treated effectively, life-sustaining support for the acutely ill or accident victim allowed lives to be saved, and even organ failure could be counteracted by machines and later transplantation. Even though the body of medical knowledge increased steadily and still continues to grow, culminating in endeavors such as the Human Genome Project, the quality of care is far less glorious. Current care can even be dangerous, and the gap between the medical knowledge and the care provided produces situations in which patients do not get what they need. This problem has been explicitly stated in two recent reports of the Committee on Quality of Health Care of the United States Institute of Medicine, "To Err is Human: Building a Safer Health System" and "Crossing the Quality Chasm: a New Health System for the 21st Century" [1,2]. These reports have been complemented by a series of publications on complexity and clinical care in the *British Medical Journal* underlining the need for a change within medical care [3,4].

Health care systems in developed countries share a common feature, which has been accentuated over the last decade. These health care systems are fragmented because of medical subspecialization, by the split between general health care and mental health care, and by the rupture between primary and secondary health care settings. Such fragmented health care systems often are not able to deliver what patients need and what standards of care recommend. An important subgroup of patients who specifically suffer from these splits in current health care systems—resulting in either its underuse or excess use—are the frail elderly, the chronically ill who have multiple morbidities (including psychiatric morbidity), those who abuse substances, and patients who have persisting functional complaints. In the following articles these patients are designated as the "complex medically ill." The report "Crossing the Quality Chasm: a New Health System for the 21st Century" is relevant to the care of these patients. It states, "Quality problems occur typically not because of failure of goodwill, knowledge, effort or resources devoted to health care, but because of fundamental shortcomings in the ways care is organized. Trying harder will not work; changing systems of care will." The report mentions six aims of quality health care. Care should be safe, effective, timely, patient-centered, efficient, and equitable. Ten new rules for achieving these aims are mentioned and contrasted with old rules (Box 1).

Complex medically ill patients are the most vulnerable to the deficiencies of a fragmented health care system and most in need of these new rules. This book is devoted to them and focuses on issues such as who these complex patients are, what kind of problems they have, how they can be conceptualized, and how new models of service delivery—including early identification, assessment, treatment planning, interdisciplinary communication, and coordination of care—can improve their situation.

George Engel called in *Science* more than 40 years ago for a biopsychosocial model of disease, which integrates somatic, psychologic, and social aspects of disease, as opposed to the medical model [5]. The relevance of the biopsychosocial model is acknowledged and supported by an impressive body of evidence; it also is reflected in the previously mentioned series of articles on complexity science in the *British Medical Journal* [3,4]:

> Human beings can be viewed as composed of and operating within multiple interacting and self adjusting systems (including biochemical, cellular, physiological, psychological and social systems). Their illness arises from dynamic interaction within and between these systems not from failure of a single component [3].

Psychiatric and somatic morbidity often coexist, and functional limitations, psychologic state, social support, and health care use are interrelated. In addition, confounding variables, such as depression or socioeconomic status, have been proven to influence morbidity and mortality of somatic diseases. Engel's vision influenced the care of patients who have chronic and life-threatening diseases and resulted in disease-management programs that integrate psychologists, social workers, and paramedics in the

---

Box 1. Rules determining patient care

Old rules
1. Care is based on visits.
2. Professional autonomy drives variability.
3. Professionals control care.
4. Information is a record.
5. Decisions are based on training and experience.
6. "Do not harm" is the responsibility of an individual clinician.
7. Secrecy is necessary.
8. The system reacts to the needs.
9. Cost reduction is sought.
10. There is preference for professional roles over the system.

New rules
1. Care is based upon a continuous healing relationship.
2. Care is customized to patient needs and values.
3. The patient is the source of control.
4. Knowledge is shared and information flows freely.
5. Decision making is evidence based.
6. Safety is a system responsibility.
7. Transparency is necessary.
8. Needs are anticipated.
9. Waste is continuously decreased.
10. Cooperation among clinicians is a priority.

---

treatment of patients suffering from diabetes, Parkinson's disease, organ failure, or cancer. Disease management, however, lacks a specific patient-tailored approach, and complex medically ill patients do not fit these programs.

In contrast to the classic disease-oriented approach, this issue focuses on a generic approach based on the concepts of case complexity and care complexity. After presenting epidemiologic, conceptual, clinical, scientific, and health care delivery aspects of the complex medical patient, different models of integrated care and ways of operationalizing complexity in clinical practice are discussed; a method for early identification and an action-oriented assessment, leading to decision support and management, as well as enhanced interdisciplinary communication, is introduced. This clinically driven but empirically based approach for the care of the complex patient has been integrated successfully in different settings.

The book addresses professionals, such as medical doctors and nurses, paramedical professionals, psychiatrists and psychologists working in the general hospital, hospital information specialists and managers, health plans/insurance companies, health care policy makers, epidemiologists, and politicians.

Frits J. Huyse, MD, PhD
Department of General Internal Medicine
University Medical Center Groningen
Hanzeplein 1, 9700 RB
Groningen, The Netherlands

E-mail address: f.j.huijse@int.umcg.nl

Friedrich C. Stiefel, MD, PhD
Service de Psychiatrie de Liaison
Centre Hospitalier Universitaire Vaudois
Rue du Bugnon 44
CH-1011 Lausanne, Switzerland

E-mail address: frederic.stiefel@chuv.ch

References

[1] Institute of Medicine. To err is human: building a safer health system. Committee on Quality of Health Care in America. Washington (DC): National Academy Press; 2000.
[2] Institute of Medicine. (2001). Crossing the quality chasm: a new health system for the 21st century. Committee on Quality of Health Care in America. Washington (DC): National Academy Press; 2000.
[3] Wilson T, Holt T. Complexity and clinical care. BMJ 2001;323:685–8.
[4] Plesk PE, Wilson T. Complexity, leadership, and management in healthcare organizations. BMJ 2001;323:746–9.
[5] Engel GL. The need for a new medical model: a challenge to biomedicine. Science 1977;196: 129–36.

ELSEVIER
SAUNDERS

THE MEDICAL
CLINICS
OF NORTH AMERICA

Med Clin N Am 90 (2006) 533–548

Assessing the Effectiveness of Integrated Interventions: Terminology and Approach

Graeme Smith, MD, BS, DPM, FRANZCP*,
David Clarke, MBBS, PhD, FRANZCP

*Department of Psychological Medicine, Monash University, Monash Medical Centre,
246 Clayton Road, Clayton 3168, Victoria, Australia*

The popular and professional response to the emerging concept of integrated medicine is similar in degree and character to that shown to Engel's biopsychosocial model of illness that was proposed in the 1960s. That model's insistence that doctors need to attend to the patient's culture, psychological being, behavior, and inner life in a systematic way had such apparent face validity that it became the guiding ethic of medical education, if not practice, for the rest of the twentieth century. This occurred despite the difficulties in operationalizing and testing the model empirically, as many investigators have pointed out [1]. The integrated medicine model, arguably a derivative of the biopsychosocial model, has had a similarly enthusiastic response that is not matched by empirical evidence for its impact on outcome for patients. The paucity of such evidence has not stopped the promotion of integrated care on ideological grounds. The biopsychosocial model survived without testing because it was proposed at the beginning of a postmodern era that was ready to accept new perspectives and deconstruction of long-held views of medical practice. It was attractive because it provided a theoretic framework for understanding difficult clinical problems—as an interaction between the body, the mind, and the social system. The context in which "integrated medicine" emerges is different; it is that created by the challenges posed by evidence-based medicine and cost efficiency. Ironically, the limitations of application of quantitative methodology to complex interventions in complexly ill patients in a complex health system has caused researchers to return to the methodology of the

* Corresponding author.
  E-mail address: graeme.smith@med.monash.edu.au (G. Smith).

biopsychosocial model—the use of the narrative account of the patient's experience of being ill and interacting with the health care system. Qualitative methodology has advanced to the stage where it provides an acceptable way of complementing data that are derived from quantitative studies, and may outstrip them in showing why it has been so difficult to translate research findings into practice [2].

Testing the hypothesis that integrated care produces better outcomes has proved difficult. The systemic factors that are involved require highly sophisticated research methodology [3,4]. Shojania and Grimshaw [5,6] observed that improvement on the modestly positive, but often conflicting, outcomes that have been reported so far in the health quality improvement field, of which integrated care is an example, can occur only if there is more rigorous research on all aspects of the process. Besides more precise definition of all terms involved, there is a need for greater conceptual understanding of complexity, clearer theoretic models and hypotheses, more detailed accounts of interventions, and better data analysis and systematic review techniques. This article reviews what we have learned so far about integrated care and its related activities, and discusses the conceptual and methodological difficulties that are impeding progress in studying its application. It is not a systematic review of reviews, but rather uses such reviews to illustrate the problems.

Terminology

Integrated medicine

In attempting to define the term "integrated medicine" it may be useful to pose the questions, "How would we recognize it if we saw it?" and "How would it differ from "nonintegrated medicine?"". When Engel developed his biopsychosocial model in the 1960s, his target of criticism was his fellow physicians, whom he believed neglected the psychological and social factors in their diagnosis and management. He pleaded for integrated care by individual clinicians. Today the prevailing language of populations and cost containment threatens achievement of this. O'Donnell [7] reminds us that "evidence-based medicine deals with populations; clinicians deal with individuals." The more complex the illness, the truer this is. Some of the current literature on integrated medicine and integrated care focuses on this wider responsibility of the clinician, particularly that on primary care and nursing, but also on other disciplines where "case management" is emphasized. "Integrated care" in this sense is recognized by the acceptance by one individual clinician of responsibility for assessment, planning, linking, monitoring, advocacy, and outreach with respect to all factors that are pertinent to meeting an individual's health care needs and achieving cost-effective outcomes [8]. Integration of biological, psychological, and social issues for that individual would be expected.

Integration of care

Another, and more prevalent, concept is that of "integration of care," the "linking" component of case management that was described above. This has become necessary because in modern medicine assessment and care have become split on the basis of organ systems, particularly for cases that are described as "complex." Furthermore, the psychological and social systems of the patient continue to be split off, despite 50 years of the biopsychosocial model [9]. Even if all relevant factors in all domains are identified, the mechanisms for linking them, planning integrated management, and monitoring its outcome often are missing. Nonintegrated care in such a case is recognizable in the despair of the patient and their family that is expressed as their inability to identify anyone who can take responsibility for the whole of the patient. An integrated care plan for complex patients is recognizable because of its inclusion of a component that describes how all relevant biopsychosocial factors will be assessed and a formulation made about why this patient has become ill in this way at this time. It also describes the way in which management will be formulated and executed, including plans for linking, monitoring, advocacy, and outreach. The person who performs the case management role is identified. The way in which the patient will be involved in this process is stated.

Thus, "integrated care" applies to the individual clinician and to the health care system in which the patient is located (or should be located—which is another issue, that of access and health care prevention). David Mechanic, credited for the introduction, with Volkart, of the relevant concept of "illness behavior" in the 1960s, has conceptualized and researched integrated care extensively since then [10]. He emphasizes the need to recognize that quality of care is a property of health systems, not just of individual clinicians. External and internal factors are important; the mobilization of consumer advocates, independent watchdog agencies, and legal and governmental bodies is required [10]. The Institute of Medicine report "Crossing the Quality Chasm: A New Health Care System for the 21st Century" [11], provides a conceptual framework of the levels of health care organization that need to be targeted in any attempt to improve patient outcome, and the intermediate targets for outcome measurement.

Complexity

"Complexity" is a term that is applied to the patient and to the care (see also the article by de Jonge and colleagues elsewhere in this issue). The parameters that are used to determine whether a patient is regarded as complex include the number of organ systems involved and the number of biological, psychological, and social domains that is considered to be making a major impact. Care is regarded as complex on the basis of the number of the types of intervention that is required and the number of disciplines that is required to make major interventions. Complex patients require complex care. Integrated care and integrated medicine is essentially about such care. Simple medical problems are managed simply, often by a general practitioner or other primary care practitioner. A complex patient may have multiple organ disease, psychiatric comorbidities, and chemical dependence and be taking multiple medications. They may have increased social disadvantage and display forms of illness behavior that challenge their care providers. Each of these elements makes the illness and the care more complex. Chronic illness almost invariably becomes complex also. Chronically ill patients usually are managed by a primary care practitioner, but usually have multiple other medical and allied health specialists. Often, complex patients are managed poorly in a nonintegrated system. The poor outcomes and high levels of health care use by these patients are driving the current interest in integrated care systems.

Associated terms

In the literature, integrated medicine and integrated care are addressed under several other headings, including "integrated intervention," "collaborative practice," "shared care," "patient-centered practice," "dual disability," "disease management," "case management," "clinical decision-making," "clinical decision rules," "care pathways," and "information transfer." The concept of screening for illness and complexity also is relevant. The diversity of terms and concepts that are in use reflects the fact that different disciplines and different levels of health care providers—and professionals outside of the health care system—have begun to approach this field. Each tends to use the theories and language of its own discipline. Fortunately, most of the systematic and other forms of review in this area allow for these synonymous or overlapping concepts, and offer a synthesis. "Quality improvement" in the health domain is the umbrella heading under which all of these topics are addressed.

Methodology of integrated care

Disappointment and frustration at the limited evidence that has emerged for the effectiveness of quality improvement in health care has prompted a focus on the methodology and theoretic underpinnings of the endeavor, and on the problems that are created by the lack of a clear definition of the concepts involved. This section reviews the definition and theoretic status of the overarching concept of disease management and of its components: disease management plans, interprofessional collaboration, screening, and case management. It also addresses the problem of choice of outcome measures. The different methodologies highlight the clash of the aims of the two cultures that are involved in health care delivery; clinical care and health care administration.

Disease management plans

Shojania and Grimshaw [5] pointed to the lack of consensus about the definition of disease management as being one of the reasons why the application of this popular concept has had such modest success when tested empirically. The authors of a major systematic review used the following definition: "An intervention designed to manage or prevent a chronic condition using a systematic approach to care and potentially employing multiple treatment modalities" [12]. The concept is broader than that of interprofessional collaboration and case management, although it usually would involve those processes. Disease management plans emphasize the use of evidence-based practice guidelines. Prevention by screening, education, and monitoring are other key components. The U.S. Government has funded several demonstration disease management projects, but such projects seem premature; further research on the conceptual model and its active ingredients is required [13]. In the U.S. Agency for Healthcare Research and Quality review on hypertension in the series "Closing the Quality Gap," Walsh and colleagues [14] highlighted the evidence for the impact of organizational change. In volume 1 of this series [15], the investigators provided an extensive review of organizational, social, and other discipline-based theories of change of the type that should underpin research that aims to demonstrate quality improvement. They argue for development of theories with greater predictive value about overcoming barriers to change (see also the article by Egede and the article by Huyse and colleagues elsewhere in this issue).

Interprofessional collaboration

Interprofessional collaboration is required in the quality improvement of health care delivery to complexly ill patients. The apparently self-evident concept of interprofessional collaboration is complex, yet there is surprisingly little theoretic consideration of the process. There is sufficient evidence that it is unrealistic to assume that it is sufficient to bring professionals together in any sort of collaboration without a theoretic framework [16]; however, doing so poses considerable challenges [17]. Interprofessional collaboration can occur at levels that differ qualitatively from each other. Interagency collaboration often involves written communication only, with no ground rules about the method of collaboration. Multidisciplinary teamwork requires only a degree of cooperation and conferring, without a defined philosophy. Transdisciplinary teams are characterized by a novel, often discipline-free, approach that requires transparency of the conceptual basis of its functioning and their interventions. Such teams are found often in nongovernment agencies. Members tend to have had training in different disciplines and have developed eclectic practices in these more flexible settings. Transdisciplinary collaboration is difficult to achieve. Western health care systems are based on autonomy of its disciplines, particularly that of doctors. Collaboration challenges this. It is important to distinguish these forms of collaboration when assessing the literature on integrated care.

D'Amour and colleagues [16] provide a review of the existing core concepts and theoretic frameworks in a supplement of the *Journal of Interprofessional*

Care that was devoted to the topic. They highlight the diversity in conceptualization. Although most investigators identify sharing as an important concept in collaboration, there is considerable diversity in what they regard as being shared: responsibility, decision-making, health care philosophy, data, and planning and intervention [16]. What seems most difficult to share is professional perspective. How can this be done without prejudicing disciplinary integrity? This applies to intradisciplinary differences as well; the difference between perspectives of the various medical specialties and subspecialties often are marked—nowhere more obvious than in the difference between psychiatry and the other medical specialties [18]. Can there truly be eclectic sharing? Eclecticism requires a sound theoretic basis, otherwise its practice cannot be evaluated critically. Transdisciplinary teams attempt this. The concepts of partnership and interdependence are relevant here, and D'Amour and colleagues [16] document the extensive consideration of them in the literature. Zwarenstein and colleagues [19] discuss the revolutionary changes in health professional education that would be required if these strong disciplinary identity forces are to be overcome. There would need to be formal courses in interprofessional collaboration. Some programs would need to aim at producing transdisciplinary practitioners, and harness the experience of those who already practice in this way.

With respect to the integrated care of complexly ill patients, a further challenge is that the team of professionals that is involved likely differs from patient to patient. These professionals constitute a team that is brought together for a specific purpose. Although the requirement to reflect on what sort of interprofessional team they are, and how they should operate is particularly great in such a case, the logistics are daunting and usually preclude it. An ongoing process of reflection that is operationalized in a way that provides such ad hoc teams with a ready framework on which to base their collaboration is required.

Collaboration is an example of group function, about which there is an extensive literature that includes psychodynamic theoretic frameworks, process theory, and systems theory [16]. Shojania and colleagues [15] provide an extensive review of organizational, social, and other discipline-based theories of change of the type that should underpin research that aims to demonstrate quality improvement. Concepts of power, leadership, responsibility, and accountability and the process of decision-making are prevalent. Many of these processes are overt in the team meetings, or are at least made so readily by a process of reflection; however, many are more subtle, and are driven by team members' unconscious processes for which the group setting provides a rich vehicle for expression. These issues were reviewed by Obholzer and Roberts [20]. Whether or not the patient is included formally in the group process, he or she is there, as an organizing focus but also as an object for projection for the unconscious processes that are at work in the group. Inclusion of the patient in the collaborative process is a major challenge, theoretically and practically.

D'Amour and colleagues [16] conclude that the limited literature shows that two elements of collaboration require attention: the construction of a patient-centered collective action that is appropriate to the complexity, and the construction of a team life that integrates perspectives and engenders trust and respect. Instruments, such as the Partnerships Analysis Tool [21], assist members of partnership groups to reflect on these tasks and to monitor the effectiveness of the mechanisms that were developed to address them. Such data form the basis for measuring the contribution of factors to the degree of collaboration, and of the effectiveness of that for better patient outcome.

Clinical decision support systems

Kawamoto and colleagues [22] define a clinical decision support system as any system that is "designed to aid directly in clinical decision-making, in which characteristics of individual patients are used to generate patient-specific assessments or recommendations that are then presented to clinicians for consideration." These systems are used most often in the management of chronic conditions, but they may have much simpler applications (eg, laboratory test reminders). Systems vary in complexity, and range from simple reminders through feedback systems to sophisticated diagnostic and management recommendations (see also the article by Lyons, the article by Huyse and colleagues, and the article by Stiefel and colleagues elsewhere in this issue). More sophisticated systems are likely to have used screening tools. Systematic reviews must attempt to deal with these differences, and the fact that descriptions of the components often lack detail.

Case management

Case management is an old concept that was revitalized in the mental health field in the 1980s and in health care generally in the 1990s as the need for cost containment and other factors favored the emergence of managed care practices. It refers to a philosophy of care and to an operationalization of that philosophy. Individuals can practice case management, as can an interprofessional system and a health care organization. Case management aims extend from better patient outcome to better profit outcome. Although the term has a self-evident meaning, it is hard to provide a precise definition. That makes it difficult to discuss conceptually and to research.

Huber [8] provides an extensive discussion of the various definitions that are available, and identifies the key features as assessment, planning, linking, monitoring, advocacy, and outreach. Huber [8] classified and discussed case management models that are found in the literature. Nursing models reflect the revolutionary shift in conceptualization of nursing toward an illness management role, which is epitomized by the development of critical pathways and other care plans, and the extension of responsibility beyond the hospital into the community. Social work models vary from that of primary therapist to brokerage and interdisciplinary team work, but the emphasis is on advocacy. General health care models include disease management, rehabilitation, and the all-embracing models of managed care and government, with their cost-containment emphasis. Some models are specifically interdisciplinary. D'Amour and colleagues [16] point out that few such models have been subjected to evaluation of their constructs.

Outcome measures

On what outcomes should we focus in exploring the efficacy and effectiveness of integrated care? Here it is important to distinguish between outcome measures that are clinical and about the patient, and process measures that concern benchmarks for health service delivery. From the patient's point of view, symptom relief, quality of life, satisfaction with the care provided, and perhaps, cost benefit are important. Family and care providers would have similar concerns. Clinicians should be concerned about the same issues, but together with the health care system involved also would focus on duration and number of admissions, number of tests, and number of services involved, because these are most pertinent to costs. At wider levels there may be interest in the cost-efficacy for the state. This is a complex matter. Is it sufficient to focus only on cost-effectiveness (ie, the ratio of monetary costs to specific treatment outcomes) or should we take into account the patient's quality of life, their productivity and role in family and community activities, and their reduced demand on other services? The latter three outcome measures are included in cost-benefit and cost-offset studies [23].

A compounding problem is that although complexity can be defined in terms of the number of organ systems and the number of health care professionals that are involved, the issues that arise depend to a large extent on the primary organ system that is involved. Thus, the literature targets patients with the most frequently occurring conditions: diabetes, coronary heart disease, stroke, renal failure, asthma, arthritis, and depression. It is difficult to pool these studies, and there may be insufficient numbers in each case to permit a meta-analysis of results [2]. Complexity also implies that patients may have disorders of more than one system; this has been addressed poorly in the literature. The methodological issues that must be addressed when performing evaluations escalate in complexity as one moves from simple outcome measures (eg, rates of readmission) to systems level outcomes. Such studies are formidable and may account for the dearth of data about the efficacy of integrated care, let alone its effectiveness (ie, its usefulness outside of the experimental setting).

There is increasing interest in the impact of integrated care projects on the development of models of interprofessional collaboration, and ultimately, on the philosophy and implementation of health care professional undergraduate and postgraduate education.

Effectiveness studies

Efficacy versus effectiveness

Most reviews of the quality improvement literature draw attention to the problems of transferring successful research-based methodology into clinical practice. Even when resistance to change and resource issues are overcome in ways that permit implementation of methods that are shown to be efficacious, their effectiveness in real-life settings often is less apparent. Shojania and Grimshaw [5,6] review the way in which we have come to this realization, the extent of the problem, and the theories that have been developed to help understand why it exists. They argue that although quality improvement, knowledge translation, and implementation research have burgeoned necessarily and become more sophisticated, there remains a need for more rigorous research on the translation of the results of systematic reviews into practice.

There is an increasingly held view that it is no longer sufficient to implement a new intervention; its impact must be evaluated because it may be producing harm. The term "health technology assessments" has been used to describe the sort of methodology that is available in the measurement of implementation of new interventions and guidelines [6]; however, resource issues usually prevent the use of randomized, controlled evaluation of implementation, which leads to the use of less rigorous techniques that may obfuscate the results. For example, resorting to simple "before and after" measures may result in confounding by unmeasured temporal changes. Although the problem of translation has been researched little, it seems that the greatest success can be expected when the active ingredients of the intervention are identified, the intervention is applied as faithfully as possible, and the setting is similar to that of the original research. Earlier reviews of strategies that aimed at increasing provider compliance with guidelines suggested that the use of multifaceted interventions was required.

Quantitative versus qualitative methodology

As will become apparent in the section that follows, the amount of evidence for the efficacy and effectiveness of integrated care that is available from systematic reviews is small, and there is considerable conflict. The small number of studies explains this in part; however, the complex nature of the interventions and of the target patients' conditions probably is more relevant. Quality improvement studies require considerable effort in identifying the right questions to ask, operationalizing the interventions, and choosing the appropriate outcome measures [24]. Usually, systematic reviews of studies performed limit themselves to quantitative data from controlled trials, and they prioritize randomly controlled trials. They may fail to retrieve important literature. Controlled trials have an important place in this field, but the questions asked also require qualitative methodology [24]. This is recognized increasingly, for instance by the Cochrane Qualitative Research Methods Group & Campbell Process Implementation Methods Group [25].

Synthesis of data

We depend on systematic reviews of studies to provide a guide as to what new interventions to implement; however, reviewing heterogenous methodologies poses the challenge of synthesis. Bravata and colleagues [24] are critical of some of the systematic reviews on quality improvement that did not use rigorous methods for defining concepts and inclusion criteria before performing the literature search. They argue that considerable conceptual work is required to formulate an appropriate question about integrated care or its associated terms and activities before the literature review begins. There may need to be extensive consultation and the use of an expert advisory group. The amount and type of data that are gathered in that preliminary exercise may require the use of novel decision analytic frameworks to identify the appropriate questions to be asked of the literature. Bravata and colleagues [24] also address the challenge of identifying the pertinent literature, and describe how groups, such as the Cochrane Collaboration, are making use of expert advisory groups to establish comprehensive databases that aim to exhaust the topic. The need for an iterative process with feedback loops is stressed.

Some systematic reviews of complex issues, such as integrated care, select studies that are so heterogenous that meta-analysis of the quantitative data that are obtained is impossible; they present descriptions in narrative, semiquantitative form. Bravata and colleagues [24] argue that even in cases when meta-analysis is possible, the techniques that were used often were too conservative. They give examples of new techniques that permit more pooling without loss of meaning. They contend that the greater use of model-based analyses may permit greater usefulness of data that already have been reported. The methodology for refining the process of synthesis of qualitative data is being developed [2]. Bravata and colleagues [24] identify several projects that are developing methods for the narrative synthesis of qualitative and quantitative data. In a major essay on reviewing complex interventions in complex situations, Pawson and colleagues [26] argue that rather than confining themselves to attempting to answer the question "What works?", reviewers should address the question of "What is it about this program that works for whom in what circumstances?". Pawson and colleagues [26] propose a method for doing this that they name "realist review," which is underpinned by a generative model of causality that focuses on mechanisms and contexts, rather than the successionist model of causality that underpins reductionist controlled trials.

Disease management

The earlier literature on disease management suggested a generally positive effect on disease control. Weingarten and colleagues [12] concluded that education, feedback, and reminders to service providers were associated with significant improvement in patient disease control, which may be mediated by the significant improvement in service provider adherence to guidelines. Education of patients, reminders to them, and financial incentives were associated with significant improvements in their disease control. The effects on patient outcome were small, except in the case of financial incentives where a larger effect size (0.44) was observed. The biggest impact of disease management was on patients who had depression, diabetes, or hypertension. The investigators were unable to compare interventions directly, mainly because many studies used more than one. Effect sizes were used as measures of difference; the investigators warned that the clinical significance of such effect sizes may be unclear. This limited their capacity to state what significant improvements would translate into in actual practice. Recent systematic reviews of reviews emphasize these concerns [15]. Shojania and Grimshaw [5] observe that although the totality of evidence supports the benefit of disease management, the benefit may be smaller than generally believed because of failure to evaluate the roles of potential effect modifiers.

Ouwens and colleagues [27] reviewed 13 systematic reviews of integrated care programs for chronically ill patients. The illnesses covered were predominantly heart failure, diabetes, rheumatoid arthritis, cardiovascular disease, stroke, and chronic obstructive pulmonary disease. The difficulty in operationalizing the definitions, aims, and outcome measures in a way that permitted valid comparisons limited their ability to reach firm conclusions, but they believe that there was evidence that integrated care programs had positive effects on the quality of care; however, the detail in the results illustrates the limits of our knowledge derived from quantitative methodology. Only 1 review reported a significant positive effect on functional health status based on meta-analysis. No significant effects on patient satisfaction and quality of life were reported. Three of the 13 reviews reported a significant positive effect on hospital readmission or length of stay. One review (on stroke) reported a significant positive effect on mortality. No significant positive effect on financial benefit was detected. Although few statistically significant outcomes were reported, the investigators emphasize that those found reflected a trend in the other reviews, and, in particular, the conclusions of the descriptive reviews. The investigators warn about uncritical application of such research results. Translating efficacy into effectiveness requires a much better understanding of the active ingredients of an intervention, as well as close attention to definitions of process and outcome.

Effectiveness of integrated primary care

There is not a sufficient number of acceptable studies of the effectiveness of shared care across the primary–specialty care interface in chronic disease management to permit a systematic analysis [28]; however, several important studies were published recently.

Katon [29] reviewed the studies that relate to the management of depression. Two studies found that psychiatrist and psychologist collaboration with primary care physicians resulted in greater improvement in depression compared with usual care and enhanced cost-effectiveness. Similar degrees of improvement with the use of nurses or care managers were reported in five studies. These findings are consistent with those of a cautious expert review [30]. Replication of these studies in a variety of settings is needed to establish the degree of generalizability. If supporting evidence emerges, it will be necessary to research the determinants of successful collaboration. It also will be necessary to research the determinants of acceptance of such plans by health care providers and their organizations, and by patients themselves. Katon [29] discussed these issues.

A subsequent report by Katon's group on a cohort of patients who had comorbid medical illness is particularly relevant to the topic [31]. In this randomized controlled trial, the collaborative management package that was used (Improving Mood—Promoting Access to Collaborative Treatment [IMPACT]) was equally effective for depressed older adults who did or did not have comorbid medical illness. Furthermore, the collaborative care also resulted in better physical functioning [32].

Effectiveness of programs for dual disability

Dual disability is a concept in the mental health field. It refers to patients who have comorbid psychiatric and drug and alcohol problems, and also to those who have comorbid psychiatric disorder and intellectual disability. Again there is a paucity of studies on the conceptual model and its active ingredients. Vanderplasschen and colleagues [33] reviewed the small amount of research literature on drug/alcohol dual disability. They concluded that there is some good evidence for retention of patients in the service, but little evidence for impact on drug and alcohol use. Program fidelity, robustness of training for interventions, administrative support, a team approach, integration in a comprehensive network of services, and a minimal level of continuity were reported to be linked to successful implementation [33,34].

Clinical decision support systems

Kawamoto and colleagues [22] performed a systematic review of trials to identify features that are critical to success. Independent predictors of improved clinical practice were automatic provision of decision support as part of clinician workflow, provision of recommendations rather than just assessments, provision of decision support at the time and location of decision making, and computer-based decision support.

Determinants of successful interprofessional collaboration

San Martin-Rodriguez and colleagues [17] provided a systematic review of the literature concerning the systemic, organizational, and interactional determinants of successful interprofessional collaboration, and the factors that impact on it (Box 1).

Impact of collaborative interventions on patient outcome

Zwarenstein and colleagues [19] identified eight major reviews of studies in which the effects of collaborative care were compared with those of standard care, and updated these by a search of recent primary literature. They

---

Box 1. The systemic, organizational, and interactional determinants of successful interprofessional collaboration

Systemic determinants
Social: sorting out discipline and gender factors
Cultural: the culture of the disciplines and more general cultural differences
Professional system: moving to a philosophy of collaboration rather than discipline autonomy
Educational system: the role of prelicensure education in breaking down the impedances noted above

Organizational determinants
Structure: shift from hierarchical to more horizontal structure
Philosophy: a range of factors related to openness are identified
Support: leadership is needed
Resources: time, space, and adequate funding are needed
Communication: transparency of the process and appropriate documentation are required

Interactional determinants
Willingness, and belief in the philosophy of collaboration
Trust in one's own professional competence and that of others
Communication skills and processes
Mutual respect, implying knowledge of and recognition of the complementariness of others' skills and knowledge

---

Data from Ref. [17].

conclude that there is evidence for the effectiveness of collaboration interventions in a range of illnesses and settings, and a range of professionals, although no formal meta-analysis was possible. Of the 14 individual studies that were regarded as sufficiently rigorous, collaborative interventions were more effective in the following areas: geriatric evaluation and management, emergency room care for abused women, screening for sexually transmitted infections, adult immunization, fractured hip care, neonatal ICU care, depression care, and simplification of medications. Theoretic frameworks and training were not necessarily involved. There was no evidence for the impact of prelicensure interprofessionalism education on patient outcome, but the methodological problems of exploring this are formidable.

Case management for complex patients in general health care

A recent systematic review of postdischarge, nurse-led management for complex patients in general health care identified 10 acceptable studies (Latour and colleagues, unpublished data). The investigators concluded that there was moderate evidence that case management has a positive effect on patient satisfaction, but it was not possible to draw firm conclusions about its impact on other outcome measures.

Summary

- Integrated care is a term that embraces several concepts, all of which imply that the target patients have complex or chronic illness.
- There is an assumption that such patients require integrated care and benefit from it.
- Attempts to test this hypothesis have produced evidence of only modest benefit, and much of the evidence is conflicting.
- Demonstration of effectiveness of integrated interventions in the clinical setting has been less convincing.
- Often, interventions are introduced uncritically and without adequate follow-up of their effectiveness.
- More rigorous research is required on definitions, theoretic constructs, outcome measures, the science of data synthesis, and translation to the clinical setting. Recent developments in theoretic constructs in these areas give promise of better answers to the question, "What works for whom in what context?".
- Qualitative methodology should form part of this research.

References

[1] Smith GC, Strain JJ. George Engel's contribution to clinical psychiatry. Aust N Z J Psychiatry 2002;36(4):458–66.

[2] Dixon-Woods M, Agarwal S, Jones D, et al. Synthesising qualitative and quantitative evidence: a review of possible methods. J Health Serv Res Policy 2005;10(1):45–53.

[3] Learmonth M. Making health services management research critical: a review and suggestion. Sociol Health Illn 2003;25(1):93–119.

[4] Ruddy R, House A. Is clinical service development simply applied evidence-based medicine? Psychiatr Bull 2005;29:259–61.

[5] Shojania KG, Grimshaw JM. Still no magic bullets: pursuing more rigorous research in quality improvement. Am J Med 2004;116(11):778–80.

[6] Shojania KG, Grimshaw JM. Evidence-based quality improvement: the state of the science. Health Aff 2005;24(1):138–51.

[7] O'Donnell M. Evidence based literacy: time to rescue the "literature". Lancet 2000; 355(9202):489–91.

[8] Huber DL. The diversity of case management models. Lippincotts Case Management 2002; 7(6):212–20.

[9] Smith GC. The future of consultation-liaison psychiatry. Aust N Z J Psychiatry 2003;37(2): 150–9.

[10] Mechanic D. Improving the quality of health care in the United States of America: the need for a multi-level approach. J Health Serv Res Policy 2002;7(Suppl 1):35–9.

[11] Committee on Quality of Health Care in America, Institute of Medicine. Crossing the quality chasm: a new health care system for the 21st century. Washington, DC: National Academies Press; 2001.

[12] Weingarten SR, Henning JM, Badamgarav E, et al. Interventions used in disease management programmes for patients with chronic illness—which ones work? Meta-analysis of published reports. BMJ 2002;325(7370):925–32.

[13] Faxon DP, Schwamm LH, Pasternak RC, et al. Improving quality of care through disease management. Circulation 2004;109(21):2651–4.

[14] Walsh J, McDonald KM, Shojania KG, et al. Hypertension care. Available at: http://www.ahrq.gov/download/pdf/evidence/qualgap3/qualgap3.pdf. Accessed November 23, 2005.

[15] Shojania KG, McDonald KM, Wachter RM, et al, editors. Series overview and methodology. Available at: http://www.ahrq.gov/download/pdf/evidence/qualgap1/qualgap1.pdf. Accessed November 23, 2005.

[16] D'Amour D, Ferrada-Vidella M, San Martin Rodriguez L, et al. The conceptual basis for interprofessional collaboration: core concepts and theoretical frameworks. J Interprof Care 2005;19(Suppl 1):116–31.

[17] San Martin-Rodriguez L, Beaulieu M-D, D'Amour D, et al. The determinants of successful collaboration: a review of theoretical and empirical studies. J Interprof Care 2005; 19(Suppl 1):132–47.

[18] Huyse FJ, Smith GC. Consultation-liaison: from dream to reality. A systematic approach to developing C–L mental health service delivery. Psychiatr Bull 1997;21:529–31.

[19] Zwarenstein M, Reeves S, Perrier L. Effectiveness of pre-licensure interprofessional education and post-licensure collaborative interventions. J Interprof Care 2005;19(Suppl 1): 148–65.

[20] Obholzer A, Roberts VZ. The unconscious at work. London: Routledge; 1994.

[21] VicHealth. The partnerships analysis tool. Melbourne: Victorian Health Promotion Foundation. Available at: http://www.vichealth.vic.gov.au/rhadmin/articles/files/Partnerships. pdf. Accessed October 17, 2005.

[22] Kawamoto K, Houlihan CA, Balas EA, et al. Improving clinical practice using clinical decision support systems: a systematic review of trials to identify factors critical to success. BMJ 2005;330(7494):765–72.

[23] Carlson LE, Bultz BD. Efficacy and medical cost offset of psychosocial interventions in cancer care: making the case for economic analyses. Psychooncology 2004;13(12): 837–49.

[24] Bravata DM, McDonald KM, Shojania KV, et al. Challenges in systematic reviews: synthesis of topics related to the delivery, organization and financing of health care. Ann Inter Med 2005;142(12):1056–65.

[25] Cochrane Qualitative Research Methods Group & Campbell Process Implementation Methods Group. Available at: http://mysite.wanadoo-members.co.uk/Cochrane_Qual_Method/index.htm. Accessed November 22, 2005.

[26] Pawson R, Greenhalgh T, Harvey G, et al. Realist review—a new method of systematic review designed for complex policy interventions. J Health Serv Res Policy 2005;10(Suppl 1): 21–34.

[27] Ouwens M, Wollersheim H, Hermens R, et al. Integrated care programmes for chronically ill patients: a review of systematic reviews. Int J Qual Health Care 2005;17(2):141–6.

[28] Smith SM, Allwright S, O'Dowd T. Effectiveness of shared care across the primary-specialty care interface in chronic disease management. Cochrane Database Syst Rev 2004;3: CD004910.

[29] Katon WJ. The Institute of Medicine "Chasm" report: implications for depression. Gen Hosp Psychiatry 2003;25(4):222–9.

[30] Evans DL, Charney DS, Lewis L, et al. Mood disorders in the medically ill: scientific review and recommendations. Biol Psychiatry 2005;58(3):175–89.

[31] Harpole LH, Williams JW, Olsen MK, et al. Improving depression outcomes in older adults with comorbid medical illness. Gen Hosp Psychiatry 2005;27(1):4–12.

[32] Callahan CM, Kroenke K, Counsell SR, et al for the IMPACT investigators. Treatment of depression improves physical functioning in older adults. J Am Geriatr Soc 2005;53(3): 367–73.

[33] Vanderplasschen W, Rapp RC, Wolf JR, et al. The development and implementation of case management for substance use disorders in North America and Europe. Psychiatr Serv 2004; 55(8):913–22.

[34] Jerrell JM, Ridgely MS. Impact of robustness of program on outcomes of clients in dual diagnosis programs. Psychiatr Serv 1999;50(1):109–12.

ELSEVIER
SAUNDERS

Med Clin N Am 90 (2006) 549–572

THE MEDICAL
CLINICS
OF NORTH AMERICA

Epidemiologic Trends and Costs of Fragmentation

Roger Kathol, MD[a,b,*], Steven M. Saravay, MD[c],
Antonio Lobo, MD, PhD[d], Johan Ormel, PhD[e]

[a]Cartesian Solutions, Inc., 3004 Foxpoint Road, Burnsville, MN 55337, USA
[b]Departments of Internal Medicine and Psychiatry, University of Minnesota,
2450 Riverside, Minneapolis, MN 55454 USA
[c]Department of Psychiatry, Albert Einstein College of Medicine, Long Island Jewish Hospital,
400 Lakeville Road, New Hyde Park, NY 11040, USA
[d]Department of Psychiatry, Universidad de Zaragoza, Hospital Clínico Universitario,
Planta 3, San Juan Bosco 5, 50009 Zaragoza, Spain
[e]Department of Social Psychiatry and Psychiatric Epidemiology, University Medical Center
of Groningen, P.O. Box 30.0019700 RB, Groningen, The Netherlands

Regardless of whether regional or national funds, social insurance groups, employers, or individuals themselves purchase clinical services, most health care systems worldwide use independent administrative and care delivery practices. These lead to separate behavioral health (used in this article to include mental health and substance abuse) and general medical evaluation and treatment, as if the two had no connection. For example, 15% of patients who have diabetes mellitus experience depression [1–3], yet in most health care environments few diabetic patients who have depression receive timely diagnosis or treatment because psychiatric assessment and intervention occur inconsistently in the medical setting [4]. Conversely, patients with diabetes being treated for depression in the behavioral health setting are rarely asked how well controlled their blood sugars are and in few are medical adherence measures included among behavioral interventions. These disconnected general medical and psychiatric treatment practices are associated with poor diabetic and depression outcomes, increased health-related service use, and impaired workplace performance [1].

Independent general medical and behavioral health administrative or business practices (eg, largely separate marketing and sales; health contracts; benefit descriptions; clinician networks and credentialing; clinical

* Corresponding author. 3004 Foxpoint Road, Burnsville MN 55337.
E-mail address: roger-kathol@cartesiansolutions.com (R. Kathol).

documentation and claims adjudication systems; medical necessity review; case and disease management; quality improvement projects; customer and provider support services; actuarial projections; and, finally, but most importantly payment pools) have grown to such a degree that these two areas of clinical practice are supported by autonomous and complex infrastructures with competing budgets [5]. Administrators who "manage" each know little about the services and mechanisms of support for services that are provided by the other. Each has developed myopic views of health care that focus on discipline-specific diagnoses, treatment, outcome measurement, and financing without considering a growing literature about the impact that comorbid medical illness has on behavioral symptoms and cost, and vice versa.

This article explores a growing literature on:

- The low frequency and the lack of effectiveness with which psychiatric illness is identified and treated using the current paradigm in which physical and behavioral health are managed independently
- The degree to which behavioral disorders influence medical and psychiatric outcomes in patients who have general medical complaints
- The effect that independent general medical and behavioral health management has on the total cost of care
- The benefits that general medical and behavioral health care integration could bring to clinical, functional, and economic outcomes

Ultimately, the article poses and attempts to address the question, "Should behavioral health become an integral part of general medical care?". Using our current understanding of the models of integrated inpatient and outpatient general medical and behavioral health services in the medical setting and the value that they bring to outcomes in patients who have concurrent physical and behavioral complaints, the answer to this question seems to be "yes."

Behavioral health disorders in the medical setting

The prevalence of behavioral disorders in the general U.S. population has been remarkably consistent at around 30% during the last several decades [6–8]. Of this population more than half (ie, 18.5% of the total) are considered to have a "clinically significant" illness in which formal intervention would be of value [9]. Although the estimated prevalence varies considerably internationally with a range from 4.3% patients in Shanghai, China, to 26.4% patients in the United States having selected World Mental Health–Composite International Diagnostic Interview [10]–identified *Diagnostic and Statistical Manual of Mental Disorders, Fourth Edition* [11] mental disorders, most countries report that 10% to 20% of their citizens have mental disorders or substance abuse for which treatment could change outcome [12].

The frequency with which common psychiatric disorders are encountered in general medical outpatients is even greater than has been reported in community samples [13–20], especially when patients present with chronic medical conditions [15,21–23]. Furthermore, some medical diseases are associated with a higher incidence of specific psychiatric syndromes than are others. For instance, patients who have respiratory and gastrointestinal illness have a higher rate of anxiety disorders, whereas patients who have back pain, multiple sclerosis, Parkinson's disease, cancer, and stroke are more likely to have depressive disorders. Patients who have some conditions, such as cardiac disease and diabetes mellitus, have a high incidence of both.

Using the Prime-MD [24], a standardized primary care behavioral health screener, 25% to 40% of general medical outpatients have a mood, anxiety, somatoform, eating, or alcohol-related disorder [18]. The percentage affected is even higher in medical inpatients, where 40% or more can be expected to have some form of behavioral disturbance [25–28]. In some populations, the frequency of psychiatric disturbances, such as delirium in patients who have experienced burns or those who are admitted to ICUs, can be greater than 60% of those admitted. If one looks at depression alone, the average prevalence has been reported to increase from approximately 5% to 10% to 15% when moving from community samples to medical outpatients to medical inpatients [29]. Given the fact that the prevalence is so high in nonmental health clinical settings, it is not surprising that more than half of mental health care is provided in the nonmental health sector [8,30–32]. Most evaluations and treatments are provided by nonpsychiatric physicians as was documented nicely by Katerndahl and Realini [33] for patients who presented with anxiety (Table 1).

Categorical affective, anxiety, somatoform, and substance-related disorders make up the bulk of behavioral health disorders that are seen in primary care clinics. Subthreshold presentations, however, are even more common and are associated with increased disability and functional impairment (Table 2) [34]. Often manifesting as unexplained somatic complaints, subthreshold disorders make up one third to one half of patients' complaints in primary care [35,36].

Medical illness in the psychiatric setting

The prevalence of medical illness in patients who have psychiatric conditions is increased for virtually all medical disease categories (Table 3) [37]. These findings have been corroborated by several other research groups [38–40]. In fact, if those with serious and persistent mental illness are assessed selectively for concurrent general medical illness, the prevalence rates for one or more illnesses are substantial (Table 4) [39].

Table 1
Types of clinicians who see patients who have anxiety disorders

	Initial	Any Visit
Medical setting	85%	49%
Primary care office		
Primary care physician	35%	35%
General internist	6%	3%
Cardiologists	6%	9%
Otolaryngologist	6%	3%
Emergency department	43%	32%
Ambulance	15%	19%
Mental health	35%	26%
Psychiatrist	22%	24%
Psychologist	13%	10%
Social worker	4%	5%
Other setting	19%	13%

Subjects may have presented to more than one site.
Adapted from Katerndahl DA, Realini JP. Where do panic attack sufferers seek care? J Fam Pract 1995;40(3):239.

No treatment and treatment delay

Several studies have reported that two thirds of patients who have behavioral health difficulties receive no treatment for their mental illness or substance abuse problems (Fig. 1) [8,9,20,30,41,42]. Nontreatment of mental illness and substance abuse is consistent throughout the world, with even fewer persons receiving treatment in the underdeveloped countries [12,43]. Of those who receive treatment, the average delay between onset of illness and treatment is 10 years although this varies based on the illness category [44,45]. For instance, the average delay between onset of illness and treatment of depressive disorders is 6 to 8 years, whereas that for anxiety disorders is 9 to 23 years [45]. Hansen and colleagues [25] reported that 39% of medical inpatients had active psychiatric illness in their hospital. Only 12% of these were referred for psychiatric evaluation and only 6% were being treated despite "free" care in the national health system of Denmark. Treatment delay is distressingly similar for the general population, minority

Table 2
Subthreshold versus categorical diagnoses in primary care

Diagnosis	Subthreshold	Categorical
Panic disorder	10.5%	4.8%
Depression	9.1%	7.3%
Anxiety	6.6%	3.7%
Alcohol	5.3%	5.2%
Substance abuse other	3.7%	2.4%

Data from Olfson M, Broadhead WE, Weissman MM, et al. Subthreshold psychiatric symptoms in a primary care group practice. Arch Gen Psychiatry 1996;53(10):880–6.

Table 3
Prevalence of medical disorders in patients who have mental health disorders

Diagnosis	Community	Mentally Ill
Hypertension	9.2%	10.0%
Heart disease	5.6%	8.8%
Gastrointestinal disease	7.6%	12.1%
Asthma	5.5%	8.5%
Diabetes	5.8%	7.4%
Malignancy	2.1%	1.5%
Respiratory	26.3%	32.8%

$P < .001$ for all.

Data from Dickey B, Normand SL, Weiss RD, et al. Medical morbidity, mental illness, and substance use disorders. Psychiatr Serv 2002;53(7):861–7.

groups, primary care outpatient clinics, tertiary care medical specialty clinics, emergency rooms, or general hospitals [46–49].

The opportunity to treat mental disorders in the general medical sector because of their higher prevalence compared to that in the community, is also hampered by a lack or effective case finding [50–52]. Effective interventions depend on accurate and timely detection, yet delays in detection and treatment are common [44] and can affect outcome adversely [53], which potentiates chronicity and worsening of the mental disorder. Case detection alone through screening is not effective in changing outcome. Evidence-based treatment also is necessary, but it occurs infrequently (see later discussion). Furthermore, the frequency and quality of intervention does not seem to be improved by educational programs for primary care physicians. Numerous studies have demonstrated that continuous medical education lectures do not change the clinician practice patterns [54,55].

While the studies above demonstrate that treatment for psychiatric conditions is hard to obtain in the medical setting, what about access to medical

Table 4
Prevalence and comparative annual cost of medical disorders in seriously and persistently mentally ill Medicaid patients

Diagnosis	Prevalence	Cost
Pulmonary disease	31%	$3306
Heart disease	22%	$2265
Gastrointestinal disease	25%	$2438
Skeletal & connective tissue disease	19%	$960
Metabolic disease	15%	$2874
Diabetes	12%	$2139
Any medical illness	75%	
Two or more medical illnesses	50%	

Data from Jones DR, Macias C, Barreira PJ, et al. Prevalence, severity, and co-occurrence of chronic physical health problems of persons with serious mental illness. Psychiatr Serv 2004;55(11):1250–7.

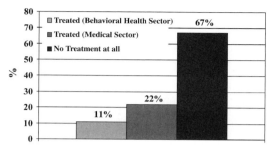

Fig. 1. Poor treatment of patients with mental illness Legend: Annually 30.5% of the population (90.3 million US citizens) has mental illness. In 58.6 million, it is moderate to severe. Thirty-three percent of those treated (8.1% of the total) receive "minimally adequate care." (*Data from* Refs. [8,9,42].)

care for the patients with mental health and substance abuse problems who have an increased prevalence of medical conditions? Are they able to access medical services that are on par with those available to patients who do not have behavioral difficulties? Several recent studies suggest that they are not [56–58]. One study suggested that even for the 50% of patients who had mental health and substance abuse disorders and an identifiable primary care physician, barriers to medical evaluation and treatment remain greater than would be expected if they had no behavioral health disorder [59]. Even preventive care is hard to obtain when a psychiatric condition is present [60].

Treatment

Numerous controlled and uncontrolled treatment trials provide support that outcomes in those who receive evidence-based treatment for most common mental illnesses, such as depression [61], are as good as or better than those for many common chronic general medical illnesses [62], such as diabetes [63], congestive heart failure [64], or arthritis [65]. Furthermore, recent evidence suggests that clinical outcomes in nonmedically ill patients can be generalized to psychiatric illness that is seen in those with medical comorbidity, although special attention is required in applying specific interventions because medical illness–based differences in treatment response, drug interactions, and adverse events that are related to treatment can occur [3,66].

The most recent survey of behavioral health disorders in the United States indicated that 32.9% of patients who have behavioral health disorders receive mental health or substance abuse care [8]. Forty-one percent of those who have "serious" disorders, 37% of those who have "moderate" disorders, and 23% of those who have "mild" psychiatric disorders are treated.

Although it is encouraging that these numbers are increasing from a similar survey that was done in the 1990s [6] and that the general medical sector is taking on a greater percentage of the behavioral health workload [8], the number of patients that receive "minimally adequate care" is substantially less than what is desired. Only 12.7% of those who receive treatment in the medical sector are given "minimally adequate care" compared with 48.3% of those who are seen in the mental health sector [67]. This fourfold difference in the administration of outcome-changing care has persisted for a decade or longer [49,68]. When you do the math, assuming that two thirds of patients who have behavioral health problems are treated primarily in the general medical sector [8,30,45], only 8.1% of those who have behavioral health disorders (12.7% of 22% treated in the general medical sector plus 48.3% of 11% treated in the behavioral health sector) receive "minimally adequate care."

Perhaps one of the most important, but least addressed, facts in providing behavioral health services to general medical patients is that even with an adequate understanding of psychiatric illness and the initiation of treatment, the outcomes with primary and specialty medical care physicians who work alone are poor. A recent summary of the literature by VonKorff and Goldberg [69] demonstrated that few outpatient treatment trials in medical patients who have depression show outcome improvement unless case management procedures are added, usually by colleagues with behavioral health backgrounds (Table 5). A part of the reason why outcomes are so poor in those in whom case management is not provided may be related to the limited number of follow-up visits that patients who have behavioral health disorders receive from general practitioners (median, 1.7 visits) when compared with their behavioral health counterparts (median, 7.4 visits) [67]. Most general practitioners do not have time to add the required education and support that are needed for depression outcome change to an already heavy clinical load.

Table 5
Outcomes of major depression in primary care studies

Study	Case management	Mental health involvement	Improved outcome
Katon, 1995	Yes	High	Yes
Katzelnick, 2000	Yes	Medium	Yes
Rost, 2001	Yes	Medium	Yes
Hunkler, 2000	Yes	Low	Yes
Wells, 2000	Yes	Variable	Yes
Simon, 2000	Yes	Low	Yes
Peveler, 1999	Yes	None	Yes
Simon, 2000	No	None	No
Peveler, 1999	No	None	No
Callahan, 1994	No	None	No
Dowrick, 1995	No	None	No
Thompson, 2000	No	None	No

Data from Von Korff M, Goldberg D. Improving outcomes in depression. BMJ 2001; 323(7319):948–9.

Interaction of general medical and behavioral health providers

Traditional models of general medical and behavioral health clinician interaction are typified by professionals with expertise in their respective disciplines (general or specialty medical versus behavioral health) using the services of those outside their discipline to address the medical or behavioral health issues for which they do not have extended training, largely on a referral basis. Once a consultation is obtained, either medical to behavioral or behavioral to medical, communication between consultant and consultee occurs only if obvious difficulties arise (eg, an adverse event, a drug–drug interaction). Further, there often is a perception that the diagnosis and treatment, particularly of behavioral health disorders, should be protected from other clinicians who are involved in the treatment of the same patient, because topics that are addressed in behavioral health are too "sensitive" for fellow medical professionals to maintain confidentiality.

Although a misinformed perception that clinical information should not be shared between general medical and behavioral health practitioners is clearly a component in noncommunication, independent general medical and behavioral health system administration also plays an important role. Despite the significant negative interaction of comorbid medical and psychiatric illness (see later discussion), there are inherent clinical (eg, time, lack of accountability for cross-disciplinary outcomes, logistics of finding the person to call), geographic (eg, separate locations, low familiarity with cross-disciplinary practitioners), and financial (eg, time-related lost income potential, incentive to care and cost shift to another reimbursement pool) disincentives for cross-disciplinary practitioners to talk with each other, far in excess of communication among other types of medical specialists.

Because the interaction of general medical and behavioral health disorders is a major factor, among others [70], which leads to poor clinical, functional, and economic outcomes, contact among those involved in the care of complex patients is essential. Lack of communication leads to the administration of ineffective or duplicative treatment, abuse of controlled substances, and drug interactions or adverse events. As importantly, it allows practitioner "splitting" and retards coordinated progress toward recovery.

Relationship of general medical to behavioral health disorders

Numerous studies now demonstrate that patients who have general medical disorders and behavioral health disorders, such as depression or anxiety, have greater morbidity associated with their medical illness, increased health care service use, and worse functional outcomes [2,23,37,39,66,71–80]. One study by Druss and colleagues [71] illustrate the impact that comorbid depression has in patients who have diabetes mellitus, cardiac disease, hypertension, and back pain in three domains (ie, clinical, economic, and functional) (Table 6).

Table 6
Healthcare use in general medical patients

	DM, CV, HT, back only (N = 1956)	Depressed Only (N = 312)	Depressed & ill (N = 100)
Health care cost	$3853	$3417	$7407
Sick days	6.64	8.79	13.48
Per capita health & disability costs	$4646	$4675	$7906

Abbreviations: CV, cardiovascular disease; DM, diabetes mellitus; HT, hypertension.

Data from Druss BG, Rosenheck RA, Sledge WH. Health and disability costs of depressive illness in a major U.S. corporation. Am J Psychiatry 2000; 157(8):1274–8.

Depression, the most common comorbid psychiatric disorder with medical illness, gets worse as medical illness severity increases but it also may contribute independently to worse medical outcomes. This association is not explained totally by poor adherence. For example, the severity of depression, ie, subsyndromal to major depression, in those who have diabetes [48], is related to worse glycemic control and hemoglobin A1c [81] levels as depressive symptoms increase [47,48]. Anxiety also has been linked with poor glycemic control [82].

Depression also predicts recurrence and mortality after myocardial infarction [83], an increased incidence of stroke in hypertensive patients [84], and doubles the mortality in patients who have strokes [85]. Several recent studies suggested that treatment with antidepressants can improve prognosis and reduce mortality in cardiovascular illnesses [86,87].

Because resolution of behavioral symptoms usually is associated with significant improvement in physical health and functionality [88–91], it is important for those who are exposed to treatment to receive interventions with the greatest likelihood of outcome change. The importance of this also is highlighted by a significant improvement in medical morbidity, especially when psychosocial and cognitive behavioral approaches are integrated with medical intervention [80,82,92], and a decrease in the total cost of care for primary care patients who receive evidence-based antidepressant therapy for depression when compared with those who do not (Table 7) [93].

Results of outcome-changing therapy are as important for restoration from disability as they are for decreasing the total cost of care (Fig. 2). These findings were replicated in two independent settings [94,95].

Data that documented high service use with poor outcomes in patients who had behavioral health problems are not limited to depression. Perhaps of greater importance is that there is an accumulating number of studies that show that intervention, especially when integrated in the medical setting, leads to significant reductions in total health care costs for patients who have anxiety disorders [77,96], delirium [97–101], substance abuse disorders [102–104], or somatization disorder [76,105–110].

Table 7
Reduced total cost at 6 months with recommended antidepressant treatment

	Minimally adequate treatment	Less than minimally adequate treatment	P
Outpatient	$1690	$1690	NS
Physical health	$1131	$1161	
Mental health	$559	$529	
Inpatient	$182	$932	.006
Mental health	$60	$147	
Physical health	$104	$785	
Total cost	$1872	$2622	.034

Abbreviation: NS, not significant.
Data from Revicki DA, Simon GE, Chan K, et al. Depression, health-related quality of life, and medical cost outcomes of receiving recommended levels of antidepressant treatment. J Fam Pract 1998;47(6):446–52.

Kathol and colleagues [5], using health plan claims on 250,000 members, showed that those who used behavioral health services (defined in their study as any patient with at least one *International Classification of Disease, Ninth Edition* [111] mental health claim [9.5% of population], chemical dependence claim [0.7%], or both [0.4%], regardless of the practitioner who made it) used nearly twice the number of health care services as did those who had medical or pharmacy service use alone (Fig. 3). These findings were similar to several other [112–116], but not all [117], studies. Only 17% of services that were used by patients who had mental illness and 31% of services that were used by patients who had chemical dependence were for behavioral health. Even pharmacy service use primarily was for nonpsychiatric medications. Yet this is a population in which little communication between general medical and psychiatric practitioners occurs.

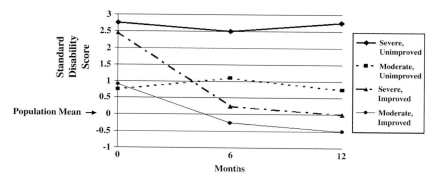

Fig. 2. Impact of effectively and ineffectively treated depression on disability. (*From* Von Korff M, Ormel J, Katon W, et al. Disability and depression among high users of health care. A longitudinal analysis. Arch Gen Psychiatry 1992;49(2):95; with permission.)

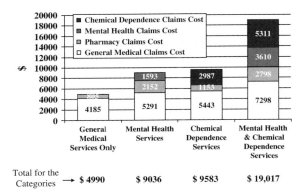

Fig. 3. 2001 claims expenditures for 250,000 members with and without behavioral health service use. (*Adapted from* Kathol RG, McAlpine D, Kishi Y, et al. General medical and pharmacy claims expenditures in users of behavioral health services. J Gen Intern Med 2005;20(2):164; with permission.)

Of special note, the few patients who used mental health and substance abuse services (patients who had dual diagnoses) had annual health care expenses that were nearly four times those of patients who did not use behavioral health services. More than half of the expenses were for medical and pharmacy services, not behavioral health care. When patients who had dual diagnoses and continuing insurance coverage were followed for an additional year, there was a stepwise decrease in the total annual cost of care for those in whom mental health and chemical dependence service needs subsided (Table 8) [5]. This suggests an association between behavioral health improvement and a reduction in total health care cost.

Table 8
Mean claims expenditures in 2001 for patients who had mental health and chemical dependence claims in 2000

	# of Patients	Annual spending per patient	Compared with average annual cost
Service use in 2000	768 (100%)	$16,634	
Service use in 2001	768 (100%)	$12,506	
Subgroups of patients in 2001:			
Well in 2001			
No mental health or chem dependence	250 (33%)	$5,729	1.5×
Better in 2001			
Mental health problems only	281 (37%)	$12,736	3.4×
Chemical dependence only	65 (8%)	$10,471	2.4×
Same in 2001			
Persistent mental health and chem dependence	172 (22%)	$22,752	5.4×

Adapted from Kathol RG, McAlpine D, Kishi Y, et al. General medical and pharmacy claim expenditures in users of behavioral health services. J Gen Intern Med 2005;20(2):160–7; with permission.

General medical and behavioral health care integration

Nonintegrated general medical and behavioral health care

In the introduction the blanket statement was made that most health systems address behavioral health and general medical needs for patients using independent administrative and business practices (Fig. 4). Although separately managed care occurs in widely divergent payment systems from country to country and even region to region, it typically leads to clinical service delivery for behavioral health that is remote from the rest of medical care. In most settings, this separation stems from segregated and fixed budgets (carve-out) or subbudgets (carve-in) for medical and behavioral health services, even when the administrative unit—whether a government agency or insurance carrier—is a single entity.

In the United States, more than 80% of patients who have medical insurance are supported for behavioral health needs by subcontracted "carved-out" behavioral health managed care companies. In the remainder, behavioral health needs are supported through a subsection of medical insurance companies (ie, "carve-ins"). The process through which behavioral health claims are paid, however, is similar for "carve-outs" and "carve-ins"; an independent subbudget that is designated specifically to reimburse behavioral health providers for behavioral health services constitutes a separate bottom line. Service use by uninsured patients in the United States (invoking a variety of public health funding pools and mechanisms) and most other countries' national health plans are handled with a variant of the "carve-in" model. For these, one overall health budget, usually with a fixed amount that is designated to cover behavioral health services and another to cover general medical services, adjudicates the health care of the population.

By now, most readers are wondering about the importance of this seemingly subtle distinction. The point that is being made is that regardless of whether one payor or two is responsible for general medical and behavioral health services, in the preponderant international health care paradigm,

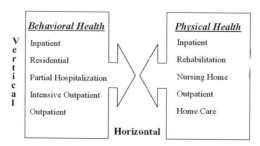

Fig. 4. A noncommunicating system. Vertical integrates care across acuity levels. Horizontal integrates care across disciplines. Both are important.

budgets and adjudication of claims are separate. Furthermore, the metrics that are used to measure quality, value, and outcomes are separate. The dynamics of this are interesting.

One of the primary objectives of Australia's First National Mental Health Plan, which was enacted in 1992, was the improved treatment of mental disorders in the primary care setting [118]. Despite a high priority, support for the section of psychiatry in Australia that is devoted to this area of practice and for behavioral health support for primary care physicians has decreased as a result because neither the mental health system nor the general medical health system wants to surrender financial resources from "their budget" to forward this clinical priority [119]. This is just one of many examples in which competing budgets interfere with care integration.

The poor clinical, functional, and financial outcomes for patients who have concurrent general medical and psychiatric illness in health systems that independently manage general medical and psychiatric practice have been discussed. In the United States, separation began in earnest in the 1980s as an attempt to curb abuse [120] and to decrease the large variances in mental health interventions. Close monitoring and restriction of "unnecessary" behavioral health services served a useful purpose for several years, and brought behavioral health treatment into closer compliance with its evidence base. Between the 1980s and today, spending on behavioral health services in the United States decreased from 8% of the health care budget to 3%. After the first several years most inappropriate care had been squeezed from the system; however, highly restrictive use review practices persisted [121].

It wasn't until 1999 that the story behind the continued restrictive behavioral health business practices was told. Until that time, widely publicized reductions in behavioral health service use—perceived cost savings to purchasers—averaged approximately 40% [122]. Savings were accomplished largely by use review practices in which "unnecessary" services [123], as determined by the managed behavioral health plans, met with payment denial.

In a simple but elegant study, Rosenheck and colleagues [114] followed total health care costs as managed behavioral health practices were introduced for factory workers of a company in the Northeast United States over a 3-year period. They were able to confirm, as in previous studies, that there was a 38% decrease in behavioral health costs. Because they measured total cost, however, they also documented a 37% increase in medical costs with a net increase of $160 per employee adjusted to 2005 dollars (Table 9). Reduced behavioral health costs merely had shifted from mental health to medical benefit expenditures. During the study, the investigators also recorded a 22% increase in absenteeism among users of behavioral health services and a 10% decrease in absenteeism in employees who did not use the services. The company that purchased independently managed behavioral health services paid more for an inferior product that also increased their disability costs.

Table 9
Behavioral health carve-outs associated with increased total annual health care costs

Introduced BH practices	BH service users	Non-BH service users
BH Expenditures	Decreased 37.7% ($1912 to $1192)	
Non-BH expenditures	Increased 36.6% ($2325 to $3175)	Increased 1.4% ($1297 to $1315)
Net total cost of care	Increased 3% ($4241 to $4369)	Increased 1.4% ($1297 to $1315)
Days absent from work	Increased 21.9% (6.4 to 7.8 days)	Decreased 10.8% (4.0 to 3.6 days)

Data from Rosenheck RA, Druss B, Stolar M, et al. Effect of declining mental health service use on employees of a large corporation. Health Aff (Millwood) 1999;18(5):193–203.

Integrated general medical and behavioral health care

Studies of inpatient and outpatient programs that integrate general medical and mental health screening and treatment have demonstrated improved outcomes [80,124–127] in comparison with other models, such as usual care or screening results provided to primary care physicians [128–130] (also see the article by Smith and Clarke elsewhere in this issue). Evidence-based data from prospective, randomized, controlled studies in primary care have demonstrated the effectiveness of integrated on-site models compared with treatment as usual in depression and panic disorder [66,68,80,96,131–136] as well as a high degree of patient satisfaction with on-site mental health treatment [135].

Similar results were demonstrated for interventions in the general hospital setting when mental health programs were integrated with the general medical team, as compared with screening alone [130,137–141] (also see the article by Smith and Clarke elsewhere in this issue). Successful integrated programs to prevent the emergence of delirium on a geriatric unit [99,100,142] also have been reported, as have preventive programs for depression in patients who had strokes [143,144]. The use of an integrated inpatient medical-psychiatric treatment model with high-acuity comorbid medical and psychiatric disorders, compared with a general medical unit, also demonstrated significantly improved outcomes [127].

Because this article suggests that handling general medical and behavioral health care independently leads to fragmented care and that care integration improves outcomes, it is important to know what is meant by integrated care. The overriding concept of general medical and behavioral health integration is deceptively simple (ie, behavioral health merely becomes an integral clinical and administrative part of general medical care). Although the concept is simple, its implementation and the process of change requires thought and effort because current systems are so entrenched in independent business practices and workflows. Some changes are clear-cut and can be done immediately, whereas others take planning. The core components of integrated care, including a stepwise progression are summarized in Box 1.

Inpatient [145–148] and outpatient [4,80,125,126,149] clinical models of general medical and behavioral health integration with evidence of effectiveness have been developed to use as guides for future clinical programs. Integrated inpatient programs are of particular interest because they address the needs of those few complex patients who use the majority of health care services (Fig. 5) [127,150].

Box 1. Core components of integrated care

Step 1 (for clinics, hospitals, and insurers)
Recognition by all staff of the interaction between medical and behavioral illness and outcomes (cultural reorientation and education)
Colocation of behavioral health and general medical staff in the general medical setting
Active collaboration and communication among cross-disciplinary and cross-trained staff (beginning shared responsibilities)

Step 2 (colocation and staff interaction in process or completed)
Proactive complex patient identification based on risk stratification or predictive modeling
A unified medical and behavioral clinical and administrative documentation system (patient record) at the clinic, hospital, and payment management levels (eg, clinical notes, coding, billing, claims adjudication)
Shared accountability for patient outcomes, medical and behavioral

Step 3
Coparticipation by all clinicians in a single provider network
A single coding, adjudication, and reimbursement system
Medical and behavioral health "medical necessity" review processes that apply to all physicians (practitioners) and for all diagnoses
Coordination of case and disease management for general medical and behavioral health disorders, especially those with complex combined illness
One payment fund for medical and behavioral health procedures and services, uniformly administered for all clinicians

---

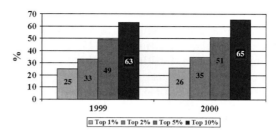

Fig. 5. Percentage of health care costs used by complex patients. (*Adapted from* Kathol R, Clarke D. Rethinking the place of the psyche in health: toward the integration of health care systems. Aust N Z J Psychiatry 2005;39:821; with permission.)

Although the value that is brought to patients occurs at the clinical level, integrated clinical programs will not be considered for creation unless the administrative support system in which they operate assures financial solvency. This means that psychiatric services, typically reimbursed at much lower rates than are medical services [151], need to be brought into conformance with their medical counterparts. From the aforementioned studies it is not difficult to see how the redistribution of funds has the potential of reaping substantial financial savings.

Insurance carriers, internationally, are coming to recognize that integrated care cannot occur when there are competing bottom lines for general medical and behavioral health services. As a result, several innovative insurers are creating integration opportunities by designing reimbursement structures that encourage clinical programs to initiate service delivery for complex comorbid patients in the medical setting [119,152–155].

Finally, although integrated care will contribute to improving psychiatric outcomes in behavioral health patients who are seen in the medical setting, it does not mean that independent behavioral health services will become obsolete. On the contrary, just as there are and will remain a need for surgicenters, ophthalmology clinics, and rehabilitation facilities, stand-alone behavioral health clinics and inpatient units will continue to serve those who have predominantly psychiatric illness. What will change is the degree to which these programs interact with the rest of medicine as they provide their services.

Summary

The data that were reviewed in this article documented that in health systems, which manage behavioral health disorders independently from general medical disorders, the estimated 10% to 30% of patients with behavioral health service needs can expect (1) poor access or barriers to medical or mental health care; (2) when services are available, most provided will not meet minimum standards for expected outcome change; and (3) as a consequence of (1) and (2), medical and behavioral disorders will be more persistent with increased complications, will be associated with greater disability, and will lead to higher total health care and disability costs than will treatment of patients who do not have behavioral health disorders.

This article proposes that these health system deficiencies will persist unless behavioral health services become an integral part of medical care (ie, integrated). By doing so, it creates a win-win situation for virtually all parties involved. Complex patients will receive coordinated general medical and behavioral health care that leads to improved outcomes. Clinicians and the hospitals that support integrated programs will be less encumbered by cross-disciplinary roadblocks as they deliver services that augment patient outcomes. Health plans (insurers) will be able to decrease administrative and claims costs because the complex patients who generate more than 80% of service use will have less complicated claims adjudication and better clinical outcomes. As a result, purchaser premiums, whether government programs, employers, or individuals, will decrease and the impact on national budgets will improve. Ongoing research will be important to assure that application of the best clinical and administrative practices are used to achieve these outcomes.

References

[1] Ciechanowski PS, Katon WJ, Russo JE. Depression and diabetes: impact of depressive symptoms on adherence, function, and costs. Arch Intern Med 2000;160(21):3278–85.
[2] Lustman PJ, Clouse RE, Freedland KE. Management of major depression in adults with diabetes: implications of recent clinical trials. Semin Clin Neuropsychiatry 1998;3(2): 102–14.
[3] Krishnan KR. Treatment of depression in the medically ill. J Clin Psychopharmacol 2005; 25(4)(Suppl 1):S14–8.
[4] Katon WJ, Simon G, Russo J, et al. Quality of depression care in a population-based sample of patients with diabetes and major depression. Med Care 2004;42(12):1222–9.
[5] Kathol RG, McAlpine D, Kishi Y, et al. General medical and pharmacy claims expenditures in users of behavioral health services. J Gen Intern Med 2005;20(2):160–7.
[6] Kessler RC, McGonagle KA, Zhao S, et al. Lifetime and 12-month prevalence of DSM-III-R psychiatric disorders in the United States. Results from the National Comorbidity Survey. Arch Gen Psychiatry 1994;51(1):8–19.
[7] Robins LN, Regier DA. Psychiatric Disorders in America. The Epidemiologic Catchment Area Study. New York: Free Press; 1991.
[8] Kessler RC, Demler O, Frank RG, et al. Prevalence and treatment of mental disorders, 1990 to 2003. N Engl J Med 2005;352(24):2515–23.
[9] Narrow WE, Rae DS, Robins LN, et al. Revised prevalence estimates of mental disorders in the United States: using a clinical significance criterion to reconcile 2 surveys' estimates. Arch Gen Psychiatry 2002;59(2):115–23.
[10] Robins LN, Wing J, Wittchen HU, et al. The Composite International Diagnostic Interview. An epidemiologic instrument suitable for use in conjunction with different diagnostic systems and in different cultures. Arch Gen Psychiatry 1988;45(12):1069–77.
[11] American Psychiatric Association. Diagnostic and statistical manual of mental disorders. Fourth edition, Text revision. Washington, DC: American Psychiatric Press; 2000.
[12] Demyttenaere K, Bruffaerts R, Posada-Villa J, et al. Prevalence, severity, and unmet need for treatment of mental disorders in the World Health Organization World Mental Health Surveys. JAMA 2004;291(21):2581–90.

[13] Ansseau M, Dierick M, Buntinkx F, et al. High prevalence of mental disorders in primary care. J Affect Disord 2004;78(1):49–55.

[14] Jackson JL, Houston JS, Hanling SR, et al. Clinical predictors of mental disorders among medical outpatients. Arch Intern Med 2001;161(6):875–9.

[15] Leon AC, Olfson M, Broadhead WE, et al. Prevalence of mental disorders in primary care. Implications for screening. Arch Fam Med 1995;4(10):857–61.

[16] Fink P, Hansen MS, Sondergaard L, et al. Mental illness in new neurological patients. J Neurol Neurosurg Psychiatry 2003;74(6):817–9.

[17] Kahn LS, Halbreich U, Bloom MS, et al. Screening for mental illness in primary care clinics. Int J Psychiatry Med 2004;34(4):345–62.

[18] Linzer M, Spitzer R, Kroenke K, et al. Gender, quality of life, and mental disorders in primary care: results from the PRIME-MD 1000 study. Am J Med 1996;101(5):526–33.

[19] Ormel J, Van Den Brink W, Koeter MW, et al. Recognition, management and outcome of psychological disorders in primary care: a naturalistic follow-up study. Psychol Med 1990; 20(4):909–23.

[20] Tiemens BG, Ormel J, Simon GE. Occurrence, recognition, and outcome of psychological disorders in primary care. Am J Psychiatry 1996;153(5):636–44.

[21] Polsky D, Doshi JA, Marcus S, et al. Long-term risk for depressive symptoms after a medical diagnosis. Arch Intern Med 2005;165(11):1260–6.

[22] Russell AS, Hui BK. The use of PRIME-MD questionnaire in a rheumatology clinic. Rheumatol Int 2005;25(4):292–5.

[23] Kessler RC, Ormel J, Demler O, et al. Comorbid mental disorders account for the role impairment of commonly occurring chronic physical disorders: results from the National Comorbidity Survey. J Occup Environ Med 2003;45(12):1257–66.

[24] Spitzer RL, Kroenke K, Williams JB. Validation and utility of a self-report version of PRIME-MD: the PHQ primary care study. Primary Care Evaluation of Mental Disorders. Patient Health Questionnaire. JAMA 1999;282(18):1737–44.

[25] Hansen MS, Fink P, Frydenberg M, et al. Mental disorders among internal medical inpatients: prevalence, detection, and treatment status. J Psychosom Res 2001;50(4): 199–204.

[26] Silverstone PH. Prevalence of psychiatric disorders in medical inpatients. J Nerv Ment Dis 1996;184(1):43–51.

[27] Arolt V, Driessen M, Bangert-Verleger A, et al. [Psychiatric disorders in hospitalized internal medicine and surgical patients. Prevalence and need for treatment]. Nervenarzt 1995; 66(9):670–7 [in German].

[28] Wancata J, Benda N, Hajji M, et al. Psychiatric disorders in gynaecological, surgical and medical departments of general hospitals in an urban and a rural area of Austria. Soc Psychiatry Psychiatr Epidemiol 1996;31(3–4):220–6.

[29] Katon WJ. Clinical and health services relationships between major depression, depressive symptoms, and general medical illness. Biol Psychiatry 2003;54(3):216–26.

[30] Regier DA, Narrow WE, Rae DS, et al. The de facto US Mental and Addictive Disorders Service System. Epidemiologic catchment area prospective 1-year prevalence rates of disorders and services. Arch Gen Psychiatry 1993;50(2):85–94.

[31] Lewis E, Marcus SC, Olfson M, et al. Patients' early discontinuation of antidepressant prescriptions. Psychiatr Serv 2004;55(5):494.

[32] Huyse FJ. From consultation to complexity of care prediction and health service needs assessment. J Psychosom Res 1997;43(3):233–40.

[33] Katerndahl DA, Realini JP. Where do panic attack sufferers seek care? J Fam Pract 1995; 40(3):237–43.

[34] Olfson M, Broadhead WE, Weissman MM, et al. Subthreshold psychiatric symptoms in a primary care group practice. Arch Gen Psychiatry 1996;53(10):880–6.

[35] Hartz AJ, Noyes R, Bentler SE, et al. Unexplained symptoms in primary care: perspectives of doctors and patients. Gen Hosp Psychiatry 2000;22(3):144–52.

[36] Kroenke K. Somatization in primary care: it's time for parity. Gen Hosp Psychiatry 2000; 22(3):141–3.

[37] Dickey B, Normand SL, Weiss RD, et al. Medical morbidity, mental illness, and substance use disorders. Psychiatr Serv 2002;53(7):861–7.

[38] Himelhoch S, Lehman A, Kreyenbuhl J, et al. Prevalence of chronic obstructive pulmonary disease among those with serious mental illness. Am J Psychiatry 2004;161(12):2317–9.

[39] Jones DR, Macias C, Barreira PJ, et al. Prevalence, severity, and co-occurrence of chronic physical health problems of persons with serious mental illness. Psychiatr Serv 2004;55(11): 1250–7.

[40] Larson MJ, Miller L, Becker M, et al. Physical health burdens of women with trauma histories and co-occurring substance abuse and mental disorders. J Behav Health Serv Res 2005;32(2):128–40.

[41] Sturm R, Sherbourne CD. Are barriers to mental health and substance abuse care still rising? J Behav Health Serv Res 2001;28(1):81–8.

[42] Alonso J, Angermeyer MC, Bernert S, et al. Use of mental health services in Europe: results from the European Study of the Epidemiology of Mental Disorders (ESEMeD) project. Acta Psychiatr Scand Suppl 2004;109(420):47–54.

[43] Ustun TB, Von Korff M. Primary mental health services: access and provision of care. In: Ustun TB, Sartorius N, editors. Mental illness in general health care. New York: John Wiley & Sons, Ltd.; 1995. p. 347–69.

[44] Christiana JM, Gilman SE, Guardino M, et al. Duration between onset and time of obtaining initial treatment among people with anxiety and mood disorders: an international survey of members of mental health patient advocate groups. Psychol Med 2000;30(3): 693–703.

[45] Wang PS, Berglund P, Olfson M, et al. Failure and delay in initial treatment contact after first onset of mental disorders in the National Comorbidity Survey Replication. Arch Gen Psychiatry 2005;62(6):603–13.

[46] Saliou V, Fichelle A, McLoughlin M, et al. Psychiatric disorders among patients admitted to a French medical emergency service. Gen Hosp Psychiatry 2005;27(4):263–8.

[47] Gross R, Olfson M, Gameroff MJ, et al. Depression and glycemic control in Hispanic primary care patients with diabetes. J Gen Intern Med 2005;20(5):460–6.

[48] Ciechanowski PS, Katon WJ, Russo JE, et al. The relationship of depressive symptoms to symptom reporting, self-care and glucose control in diabetes. Gen Hosp Psychiatry 2003; 25(4):246–52.

[49] Saravay SM. Psychiatric interventions in the medically ill. Outcome and effectiveness research. Psychiatric Clin North Am 1996;19(3):467–80.

[50] Fink P, Ornbol E, Huyse FJ, et al. A brief diagnostic screening instrument for mental disturbances in general medical wards. J Psychosom Res 2004;57(1):17–24.

[51] de Jonge P, Hoogervorst EL, Huyse FJ, et al. INTERMED: a measure of biopsychosocial case complexity: one year stability in multiple sclerosis patients. Gen Hosp Psychiatry 2004; 26(2):147–52.

[52] De Jonge P, Bauer I, Huyse FJ, et al. Medical inpatients at risk of extended hospital stay and poor discharge health status: detection with COMPRI and INTERMED. Psychosom Med 2003;65(4):534–41.

[53] Kishi Y, Meller WH, Kathol RG, et al. Factors affecting the relationship between the timing of psychiatric consultation and general hospital length of stay. Psychosomatics 2004;45(6):470–6.

[54] Lin EH, Simon GE, Katzelnick DJ, et al. Does physician education on depression management improve treatment in primary care? J Gen Intern Med 2001;16(9):614–9.

[55] Katon W, Von Korff M, Lin E, et al. Population-based care of depression: effective disease management strategies to decrease prevalence. Gen Hosp Psychiatry 1997;19(3):169–78.

[56] Salsberry PJ, Chipps E, Kennedy C. Use of general medical services among Medicaid patients with severe and persistent mental illness. Psychiatr Serv 2005;56(4):458–62.

[57] Cradock-O'Leary J, Young AS, Yano EM, et al. Use of general medical services by VA patients with psychiatric disorders. Psychiatr Serv 2002;53(7):874–8.

[58] Koran LM, Sheline Y, Imai K, et al. Medical disorders among patients admitted to a public-sector psychiatric inpatient unit. Psychiatr Serv 2002;53(12):1623–5.

[59] Levinson Miller C, Druss BG, Dombrowski EA, et al. Barriers to primary medical care among patients at a community mental health center. Psychiatr Serv 2003;54(8):1158–60.

[60] Carney CP, Allen J, Doebbeling BN. Receipt of clinical preventive medical services among psychiatric patients. Psychiatr Serv 2002;53(8):1028–30.

[61] Wells KB, Sherbourne C, Schoenbaum M, et al. Impact of disseminating quality improvement programs for depression in managed primary care: a randomized controlled trial. JAMA 2000;283(2):212–20.

[62] US Department of Health and Human Services. Mental health: a report of the Surgeon General. Rockville: US Department of Health and Human Services, Substance Abuse and Mental Health Services Administration, Center for Mental Health Services, National Institutes of Health, National Institute of Mental Health; 1999.

[63] Norris SL, Nichols PJ, Caspersen CJ, et al. The effectiveness of disease and case management for people with diabetes. A systematic review. Am J Prev Med 2002;22(4 Suppl): 15–38.

[64] Roglieri JL, Futterman R, McDonough KL, et al. Disease management interventions to improve outcomes in congestive heart failure. Am J Manag Care 1997;3(12):1831–9.

[65] Lorig KR, Ritter P, Stewart AL, et al. Chronic disease self-management program: 2-year health status and health care utilization outcomes. Med Care 2001;39(11):1217–23.

[66] Roy-Byrne P, Stein MB, Russo J, et al. Medical illness and response to treatment in primary care panic disorder. Gen Hosp Psychiatry 2005;27(4):237–43.

[67] Wang PS, Lane M, Olfson M, et al. Twelve-month use of mental health services in the United States: results from the National Comorbidity Survey Replication. Arch Gen Psychiatry 2005;62(6):629–40.

[68] Schulberg HC, Block MR, Madonia MJ, et al. Treating major depression in primary care practice. Eight-month clinical outcomes. Arch Gen Psychiatry 1996;53(10):913–9.

[69] Von Korff M, Goldberg D. Improving outcomes in depression. BMJ 2001;323(7319): 948–9.

[70] Neeleman J, Bijl R, Ormel J. Neuroticism, a central link between somatic and psychiatric morbidity: path analysis of prospective data. Psychol Med 2004;34(3):521–31.

[71] Druss BG, Rosenheck RA, Sledge WH. Health and disability costs of depressive illness in a major US corporation. Am J Psychiatry 2000;157(8):1274–8.

[72] Luber MP, Hollenberg JP, Williams-Russo P, et al. Diagnosis, treatment, comorbidity, and resource utilization of depressed patients in a general medical practice. Int J Psychiatry Med 2000;30(1):1–13.

[73] Kessler RC, Berglund P, Demler O, et al. The epidemiology of major depressive disorder: results from the National Comorbidity Survey Replication (NCS-R). JAMA 2003;289(23): 3095–105.

[74] Stewart WF, Ricci JA, Chee E, et al. Cost of lost productive work time among US workers with depression. JAMA 2003;289(23):3135–44.

[75] Sokal J, Messias E, Dickerson FB, et al. Comorbidity of medical illnesses among adults with serious mental illness who are receiving community psychiatric services. J Nerv Ment Dis 2004;192(6):421–7.

[76] Smith GR Jr, Monson RA, Ray DC. Psychiatric consultation in somatization disorder. A randomized controlled study. N Engl J Med 1986;314(22):1407–13.

[77] Salvador-Carulla L, Segui J, Fernandez-Cano P, et al. Costs and offset effect in panic disorders. Br J Psychiatry Suppl 1995;(27):23–8.

[78] Kroenke K. Patients presenting with somatic complaints: epidemiology, psychiatric comorbidity and management. Int J Methods Psychiatr Res 2003;12(1):34–43.

[79] Callahan EJ, Jaen CR, Crabtree BF, et al. The impact of recent emotional distress and diagnosis of depression or anxiety on the physician-patient encounter in family practice. J Fam Pract 1998;46(5):410–8.

[80] Katon WJ, Von Korff M, Lin EH, et al. The Pathways Study: a randomized trial of collaborative care in patients with diabetes and depression. Arch Gen Psychiatry 2004;61(10): 1042–9.

[81] Katon W, von Korff M, Ciechanowski P, et al. Behavioral and clinical factors associated with depression among individuals with diabetes. Diabetes Care 2004;27(4):914–20.

[82] Lustman PJ, Anderson RJ, Freedland KE, et al. Depression and poor glycemic control: a meta-analytic review of the literature. Diabetes Care 2000;23(7):934–42.

[83] Glassman AH, Shapiro PA. Depression and the course of coronary artery disease. Am J Psychiatry 1998;155(1):4–11.

[84] Simonsick EM, Wallace RB, Blazer DG, et al. Depressive symptomatology and hypertension-associated morbidity and mortality in older adults. Psychosom Med 1995;57(5): 427–35.

[85] Morris PL, Robinson RG, Andrzejewski P, et al. Association of depression with 10-year poststroke mortality. Am J Psychiatry 1993;150(1):124–9.

[86] Glassman AH. Does treating post-myocardial infarction depression reduce medical mortality? Arch Gen Psychiatry 2005;62(7):711–2.

[87] Rasmussen A, Lunde M, Poulsen DL, et al. A double-blind, placebo-controlled study of sertraline in the prevention of depression in stroke patients. Psychosomatics 2003;44(3): 216–21.

[88] Callahan CM, Kroenke K, Counsell SR, et al. Treatment of depression improves physical functioning in older adults. J Am Geriatr Soc 2005;53(3):367–73.

[89] Lin EH, Katon W, Von Korff M, et al. Effect of improving depression care on pain and functional outcomes among older adults with arthritis: a randomized controlled trial. JAMA 2003;290(18):2428–9.

[90] Lustman PJ, Griffith LS, Freedland KE, et al. Cognitive behavior therapy for depression in type 2 diabetes mellitus. A randomized, controlled trial. Ann Intern Med 1998;129(8): 613–21.

[91] Simon GE, Chisholm D, Treglia M, et al. Course of depression, health services costs, and work productivity in an international primary care study. Gen Hosp Psychiatry 2002;24(5): 328–35.

[92] Delamater AM, Jacobson AM, Anderson B, et al. Psychosocial therapies in diabetes: report of the Psychosocial Therapies Working Group. Diabetes Care 2001;24(7):1286–92.

[93] Revicki DA, Simon GE, Chan K, et al. Depression, health-related quality of life, and medical cost outcomes of receiving recommended levels of antidepressant treatment. J Fam Pract 1998;47(6):446–52.

[94] Von Korff M, Ormel J, Katon W, et al. Disability and depression among high utilizers of health care. A longitudinal analysis. Arch Gen Psychiatry 1992;49(2):91–100.

[95] Ormel J, Von Korff M, Van den Brink W, et al. Depression, anxiety, and social disability show synchrony of change in primary care patients. Am J Public Health 1993;83(3):385–90.

[96] Katon WJ, Roy-Byrne P, Russo J, et al. Cost-effectiveness and cost offset of a collaborative care intervention for primary care patients with panic disorder. Arch Gen Psychiatry 2002; 59(12):1098–104.

[97] Lundstrom M, Edlund A, Karlsson S, et al. A multifactorial intervention program reduces the duration of delirium, length of hospitalization, and mortality in delirious patients. J Am Geriatr Soc 2005;53(4):622–8.

[98] Naughton BJ, Saltzman S, Ramadan F, et al. A multifactorial intervention to reduce prevalence of delirium and shorten hospital length of stay. J Am Geriatr Soc 2005;53(1):18–23.

[99] Marcantonio ER, Flacker JM, Wright RJ, et al. Reducing delirium after hip fracture: a randomized trial. J Am Geriatr Soc 2001;49(5):516–22.

[100] Inouye SK, Bogardus ST Jr, Williams CS, et al. The role of adherence on the effectiveness of nonpharmacologic interventions: evidence from the delirium prevention trial. Arch Intern Med 2003;163(8):958–64.

[101] Tabet N, Hudson S, Sweeney V, et al. An educational intervention can prevent delirium on acute medical wards. Age Ageing 2005;34(2):152–6.

[102] Weisner C, Mertens J, Parthasarathy S, et al. Integrating primary medical care with addiction treatment: a randomized controlled trial. JAMA 2001;286(14):1715–23.

[103] Parthasarathy S, Mertens J, Moore C, et al. Utilization and cost impact of integrating substance abuse treatment and primary care. Med Care 2003;41(3):357–67.

[104] Holder HD, Blose JO. The reduction of health care costs associated with alcoholism treatment: a 14-year longitudinal study. J Stud Alcohol 1992;53(4):293–302.

[105] Kashner TM, Rost K, Cohen B, et al. Enhancing the health of somatization disorder patients. Effectiveness of short-term group therapy. Psychosomatics 1995;36(5):462–70.

[106] Rost K, Kashner TM, Smith RG Jr. Effectiveness of psychiatric intervention with somatization disorder patients: improved outcomes at reduced costs. Gen Hosp Psychiatry 1994; 16(6):381–7.

[107] Smith GR Jr, Rost K, Kashner TM. A trial of the effect of a standardized psychiatric consultation on health outcomes and costs in somatizing patients. Arch Gen Psychiatry 1995; 52(3):238–43.

[108] Toft T. Managing patients with functional somatic symptoms in general practice. Aarhus, Denmark: University of Aarhus; 2004.

[109] Morriss R, Gask L, Ronalds C, et al. Cost-effectiveness of a new treatment for somatized mental disorder taught to GPs. Fam Pract 1998;15(2):119–25.

[110] Hiller W, Fichter MM, Rief W. A controlled treatment study of somatoform disorders including analysis of healthcare utilization and cost-effectiveness. J Psychosom Res 2003; 54(4):369–80.

[111] National Center for Health Statistics (NCHS)/Centers for Medicare and Medicaid Services. International Classification of Diseases, Ninth Revision, Clinical Modification. Washington, DC: Centers for Disease Control and Prevention/National Center for Health Statistics; 2005.

[112] Harlow K, Johnson R, Callen P. Comparison of physical health benefits utilization. Mental and physical health claimants, 1989 and 1990. J Occup Med 1993;35(3):275–81.

[113] Simon GE, Unutzer J. Health care utilization and costs among patients treated for bipolar disorder in an insured population. Psychiatr Serv 1999;50(10):1303–8.

[114] Rosenheck RA, Druss B, Stolar M, et al. Effect of declining mental health service use on employees of a large corporation. Health Aff (Millwood) 1999;18(5):193–203.

[115] Trudeau JV, Deitz DK, Cook RF. Utilization and cost of behavioral health services: employee characteristics and workplace health promotion. J Behav Health Serv Res 2002;29(1):61–74.

[116] Thomas MR, Waxmonsky JA, Gabow PA, et al. Prevalence of psychiatric disorders and costs of care among adult enrollees in a Medicaid HMO. Psychiatr Serv 2005;56(11): 1394–401.

[117] Cuffel BJ, Goldman W, Schlesinger H. Does managing behavioral health care services increase the cost of providing medical care? J Behav Health Serv Res 1999;26(4): 372–80.

[118] Australian Health Ministers. Mental Health Statement of Rights and Responsibilities. Canberra (Australia): Australian Government Publishing Service; 1992.

[119] Kathol R, Clarke D. Rethinking the place of the psyche in health: toward the integration of healthcare systems. Aust N Z J Psychiatry 2005;39:826–35.

[120] Sharkey J. Bedlam: greed, profiteering, and fraud in a mental health system gone crazy. New York: St. Martin's Press; 1994.

[121] HayGroup. Health care plan design and cost trends: 1988 through 1998. Arlington (VA): Haygroup; 1999.

[122] Goldman W, McCulloch J, Sturm R. Costs and use of mental health services before and after managed care. Health Aff (Millwood) 1998;17(2):40–52.

[123] Grazier KL, Eselius LL. Mental health carve-outs: effects and implications. Med Care Res Rev 1999;56(Suppl 2):37–59.

[124] Yeung A, Kung WW, Chung H, et al. Integrating psychiatry and primary care improves acceptability to mental health services among Chinese Americans. Gen Hosp Psychiatry 2004;26(4):256–60.

[125] Kates N, Craven M. Shared mental health care. Update from the Collaborative Working Group of the College of Family Physicians of Canada and the Canadian Psychiatric Association. Can Fam Physician 2002;48:853–5, 859–61.

[126] Oxman TE, Dietrich AJ, Williams JW Jr, et al. A three-component model for reengineering systems for the treatment of depression in primary care. Psychosomatics 2002;43(6):441–50.

[127] Kishi Y, Kathol RG. Integrating medical and psychiatric treatment in an inpatient medical setting. The type IV program. Psychosomatics 1999;40(4):345–55.

[128] Katon W, Gonzales J. A review of randomized trials of psychiatric consultation-liaison studies in primary care. Psychosomatics 1994;35(3):268–78.

[129] Saravay SM, Strain JJ. APM Task Force on Funding Implications of Consultation-Liaison Outcome Studies. Special series introduction: a review of outcome studies. Psychosomatics 1994;35(3):227–32.

[130] Saravay S. Intervention studies in general hospital patients. In: Blumenfield M, Strain JJ, editors. Psychosomatic medicine. Philadelphia: Lippincott Williams and Wilkins; 2006.

[131] Upshur CC. Crossing the divide: primary care and mental health integration. Adm Policy Ment Health 2005;32(4):341–55.

[132] Unutzer J, Katon W, Callahan CM, et al. Collaborative care management of late-life depression in the primary care setting: a randomized controlled trial. JAMA 2002; 288(22):2836–45.

[133] Craske MG, Roy-Byrne P, Stein MB, et al. Treating panic disorder in primary care: a collaborative care intervention. Gen Hosp Psychiatry 2002;24(3):148–55.

[134] Katon W, Von Korff M, Lin E, et al. Stepped collaborative care for primary care patients with persistent symptoms of depression: a randomized trial. Arch Gen Psychiatry 1999; 56(12):1109–15.

[135] Katon W, Robinson P, Von Korff M, et al. A multifaceted intervention to improve treatment of depression in primary care. Arch Gen Psychiatry 1996;53(10):924–32.

[136] Katon W, Von Korff M, Lin E, et al. Collaborative management to achieve treatment guidelines. Impact on depression in primary care. JAMA 1995;273(13):1026–31.

[137] Levenson JL, Hamer RM, Rossiter LF. A randomized controlled study of psychiatric consultation guided by screening in general medical inpatients. Am J Psychiatry 1992; 149(5):631–7.

[138] Levitan SJ, Kornfeld DS. Clinical and cost benefits of liaison psychiatry. Am J Psychiatry 1981;138(6):790–3.

[139] Strain JJ, Lyons JS, Hammer JS, et al. Cost offset from a psychiatric consultation-liaison intervention with elderly hip fracture patients. Am J Psychiatry 1991;148(8):1044–9.

[140] Slaets JP, Kauffmann RH, Duivenvoorden HJ, et al. A randomized trial of geriatric liaison intervention in elderly medical inpatients. Psychosom Med 1997;59(6):585–91.

[141] de Jonge P, Latour CH, Huyse FJ. Implementing psychiatric interventions on a medical ward: effects on patients' quality of life and length of hospital stay. Psychosom Med 2003;65(6):997–1002.

[142] Inouye SK, Bogardus ST Jr, Charpentier PA, et al. A multicomponent intervention to prevent delirium in hospitalized older patients. N Engl J Med 1999;340(9):669–76.

[143] Wiart L, Petit H, Joseph PA, et al. Fluoxetine in early poststroke depression: a double-blind placebo-controlled study. Stroke 2000;31(8):1829–32.

[144] Jorge RE, Robinson RG, Arndt S, et al. Mortality and poststroke depression: a placebo-controlled trial of antidepressants. Am J Psychiatry 2003;160(10):1823–9.

[145] Kathol RG, Harsch HH, Hall RC, et al. Categorization of types of medical/psychiatry units based on level of acuity. Psychosomatics 1992;33(4):376–86.

[146] Kathol R, Stoudemire A. Strategic integration of inpatient and outpatient medical-psychiatry services. In: JR WMR, editor. The textbook of consultation-liaison psychiatry. 2nd edition. Washington, DC: APPI Press; 2002. p. 995–1014.

[147] Gitlin DF, Levenson JL, Lyketsos CG. Psychosomatic medicine: a new psychiatric subspecialty. Acad Psychiatry 2004;28(1):4–11.

[148] Diefenbacher A. Consultation-liaison psychiatry in Germany. Adv Psychosom Med 2004; 26:1–19.

[149] Katon W, Russo J, Von Korff M, et al. Long-term effects of a collaborative care intervention in persistently depressed primary care patients. J Gen Intern Med 2002;17(10):741–8.

[150] Deloitte & Touche. Health care service use by a small percentage of covered population–client report. 2002.

[151] Olson J. Quality, cost and impact on other needs are concerns. St. Paul (MN): Pioneer Press; 2005.

[152] Lester H, Glasby J, Tylee A. Integrated primary mental health care: threat or opportunity in the new NHS? Br J Gen Pract 2004;54(501):285–91.

[153] Grazier KL, Hegedus AM, Carli T, et al. Integration of behavioral and physical health care for a Medicaid population through a public-public partnership. Psychiatr Serv 2003;54(11): 1508–12.

[154] Kathol RG. Integrated general medical and psychiatric care: Minnesota takes the lead. Minn Med 2004;87(8):44–6.

[155] Miller J. Big picture. Managed Healthcare Executive 2005. Available at: http://www.managedhealthcareexecutive.com/mhe/article/articledetail.jsp?id=164255. Accessed June 2006.

ELSEVIER
SAUNDERS

THE MEDICAL
CLINICS
OF NORTH AMERICA

Med Clin N Am 90 (2006) 573–591

The Metabolic Syndrome, Depression, and Cardiovascular Disease: Interrelated Conditions that Share Pathophysiologic Mechanisms

Rijk O.B. Gans, MD, PhD

University Medical Center Groningen, Hanzeplein 1 9700 RB, Groningen, The Netherlands

The metabolic syndrome

The concept of the metabolic syndrome has existed for at least 80 years [1]. It was first described in the 1920s by Kylin, a Swedish physician, who noted a clustering of hypertension, hyperglycemia, and gout. Next, the concept of upper-body adiposity (android or male-type obesity, as opposed to female-type obesity) was recognized as the obesity phenotype that was commonly associated with the metabolic abnormalities associated with type 2 diabetes and cardiovascular disease. In 1988 Reaven described insulin resistance as the central feature of syndrome X, a constellation of hyperglycemia, hypertension, low high-density lipoprotein cholesterol levels, and elevated very-low-density lipoprotein triglyceride levels. More recently, the term "metabolic syndrome" (visceral obesity, dyslipidemia, hyperglycemia, and hypertension) was coined, mostly because its clinical phenotype, foremost an increase in waist circumference, helps identify individuals who are at increased risk for type 2 diabetes and cardiovascular disease.

Several sets of diagnostic criteria with different cut-off values for waist circumference, blood pressure, glucose, high-density lipoprotein cholesterol levels, and triglycerides have been, proposed by various medical societies. The International Diabetes Federation recently proposed a worldwide definition that incorporates ethnic-specific waist circumference cut-off values [2]. It should be realized, however, that the concept of the metabolic syndrome as a medical diagnosis is under debate, largely because this cluster

---

E-mail address: r.o.b.gans@int.umcg.nl

doi:10.1016/j.mcna.2006.05.002   *medical.theclinics.com*

of metabolic abnormalities and cardiovascular risk factors lacks a definitive single or major unifying pathophysiologic process, and treatment of the syndrome does not different from treatment of its components [3]. Nonetheless, this clustering of closely related cardiovascular risk factors has been focus of much interest because of its putative association with cardiovascular disease and diabetes and also with a vast array of other diseases, including cancer, schizophrenia, and depression (Box 1).

Box 1. The metabolic syndrome: changes associated with insulin resistance

Lifestyle
Cigarette smoking
Sedentary behavior

Lipoproteins
Increased free fatty acids
Increased apolipoprotein B
Decreased apolipoprotein A-1
Small, dense low-density lipoprotein and high-density lipoprotein
Increased apolipoprotein C-III

Prothrombotic
Increased fibrinogen
Increased plasminogen activator inhibitor 1
Increased viscosity

Inflammatory markers
Increased white blood cell count
Increased interleukin 6
Increased tumor necrosis factor
Increased resistin
Increased C-reactive protein
Decreased adiponectin

Vascular
Microalbuminuria
Increased asymmetric dimethylarginine
Increased uric acid
Increased homocysteine

Adapted from Eckel RH, Grundy SM, Zimmet PZ. The metabolic syndrome. Lancet 2005;365:1420.

Relationship of metabolic syndrome with cardiovascular disease,
type 2 diabetes, and depression

The metabolic syndrome is associated with an increased risk of both diabetes and cardiovascular disease. This association is not surprising because the definition of the syndrome comprises established risk factors for diabetes and cardiovascular disease. For cardiovascular disease, the relative hazard ratios range from 2 to 5 [1]. The risk of diabetes is substantial also. The cumulative incidence of diabetes in subjects with impaired glucose tolerance (and obesity) who participated in the diabetes prevention studies was approximately 30% after 3 years of follow-up [4].

A large body of evidence supports an association between type 2 diabetes, cardiovascular disease, and, recently, metabolic syndrome and the occurrence of depression. Individuals who have diabetes are twice as likely to develop depression as individuals who do not have diabetes. Interestingly, one study indicated an increased risk of depression in type 2 diabetes only when comorbid cardiovascular diseases were present [5]. The prevalence of metabolic syndrome among women who have a history of depression is twice as high as that among women who have no history of depression [6]. If one accepts obesity as a surrogate marker of the metabolic syndrome, a potential gender difference may exist. In women in the United States, obesity increases the risk of being diagnosed with major depression by 37%, whereas obese men have a 37% lower risk of depression than men of normal weight [7]. Conversely, depression is associated with an increased incidence of diabetes, which in turn seems to be mediated largely through central adiposity [8]. When depression complicates diabetes, it is significantly associated with nonadherence to medication and self-care recommendations, poor metabolic control, and, thus, increased odds of having diabetic and cardiovascular complications (see the article by Egede in this issue).

Depressed patients who do not have overt diabetes also have an increased relative risk for developing cardiovascular complications that varies between 1.5 and 2.7 depending on the magnitude of depressive symptoms [9]. Notably, also in the absence of predefined psychiatric diagnoses as major depression, psychologic factors (especially when occurring in combination) result in an increased risk for cardiovascular complications are to the risks associated with hypercholesterolemia, hypertension, and other major risk factors [10,11].

Others have postulated that there might exist a subtype of vascular depression in which cerebrovascular disease predisposes, precipitates, or perpetuates a depressive syndrome [12].

A life-course approach

The aforementioned relationships are derived largely from conventional epidemiologic studies that merely studied classic disease models (eg, smoking or obesity) as exponents of adult lifestyle that turned out to be modifiable risk factors for cardiovascular disease and diabetes. This epidemiologic approach, however, does not acknowledge many other observations that do not fit such a simple disease model. Throughout life various biologic, psychologic, and social factors act independently, cumulatively, and interactively on health and disease in adult life (Fig. 1). In a life-course epidemiologic approach the risk of disease is related to physical and social exposures during gestation, childhood, and adolescence as well as during later adult life [13].

The importance of the temporal relationships between these exposures is underscored by the existence of so-called "critical periods." For example, studies have shown that poor growth in utero relates to cardiovascular disease, type 2 diabetes, and insulin resistance in adult life. Moreover, this relationship is particularly strong or is observed only in subjects who become obese in childhood, adulthood, or both [14–16]. This finding suggests that fetal exposure may alter the metabolic system permanently but is still under influence of exposures acting later in life. Likewise, a relationship between low birth weight and psychologic distress in adult life has been documented [17].

The life-course approach also incorporates and integrates social risk processes. Socially patterned exposures during childhood, adolescence, and early adult life have been shown to influence adult disease risk and socioeconomic status (SES) [18]. SES is characterized as a composite of factors such as occupational status, economic resources, education, and social status. Longitudinal studies have indicated a strong inverse gradient between SES level and adverse cardiac events. Low SES is accompanied by poorer health habits and higher frequencies of coronary risk factors and, as would be

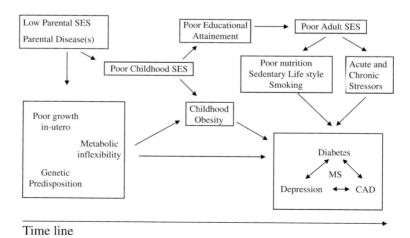

Fig. 1. Biologic and psychosocial exposures across the life timeline that influence the metabolic syndrome. CAD, coronary artery disease; MS, Metabolic Syndrome; SES, socioeconomic status.

expected, is associated with an increased prevalence of the metabolic syndrome [19,20]. At the same time, low SES is considered a chronic stressor, and persons who have low SES also have higher frequencies of mental disorders (ie, anxiety and depression) [21].

Accumulation of risk is another concept that plays a pivotal role in the life-course model of chronic diseases. More than 80 years ago Selye [22] recognized that the physiologic systems activated by stress can protect and restore but also can damage the body. To understand this paradox, the concept of allostasis has been introduced [23]. Allostasis is defined as the ability to achieve stability through change. The price of this accommodation to stress has been defined as the allostatic load [23]. It follows that acute stress (eg, the "fright, flight or fight" response or major life events) and chronic stress (the cumulative load of minor, day-to-day stresses) can add to the allostatic load and have long-term consequences. Subacute stress is defined as an accumulation of stressful life events over a duration of months and includes emotional factors such as hostility and anger as well as affective disorders such as major depression and anxiety disorders. Chronic stressors include factors such as low social support, low SES, work stress, marital stress, and caregiver strain and present as feelings of fatigue, lack of energy, irritability, and demoralization. The life-course approach is complementary to this concept and argues that factors that raise the risk of disease or promote good health may accumulate gradually over the life course, although their effects may have greater impact on later health at specific developmental periods than at other times [13].

Pathophysiologic mechanisms

To integrate biologic and psychosocial pathways, the life-course approach requires understanding the natural history and physiologic trajectory of normal biologic systems, including the brain, and how these systems are affected by chronic exposure to disease risks.

Normal stress response

As stated previously, the response of the body to maintain its stability in the face of a challenge (eg, infection or an instable social situation) comprises the allostatic response. The brain plays a pivotal role in the maintenance of body homeostasis [23]. For this purpose the brain has two avenues of communication: hormones and neurons. The sensory organs inform the brain about the external environment. The state of the internal environment is reported to the spinal cord and brain stem through feedback from virtually all organs [24]. In addition, the brain integrates information about circulating hormone and substrate availability through receptors located in areas where the blood–brain barrier allows this information to be passed to the brain. Processing of internal and external stress stimuli results in responses of the autonomic nervous system, the hypothalamus-pituitary-adrenal (HPA) axis, and the cardiovascular, metabolic, and immune systems.

The immune system is characterized by two components, the innate and the acquired immune systems. In general, the innate and the acquired immune systems react to pathogens and other antigens with an inflammatory response that, if severe enough, may include an acute-phase response as well as the formation of an immunologic memory. Fever is an example of the neuroendocrine changes that characterize the acute-phase response. Other clinical manifestations reflect complex interactions among cytokines, the HPA axis, and other components of the neuroendocrine system. The behavioral changes that often accompany this response (eg, anorexia, somnolence, lethargy, irritability, depressed mood, and social withdrawal) also reflect responses to cytokines. The HPA axis and the autonomic nervous system contain the acute-phase response and dampen cellular immunity. In addition, inflammatory input to the hypothalamus activates a reflexive, fast, and subconscious anti-inflammatory response (which until recently was unknown) through the efferent vagal nerve [25]. Vagal cholinergic activation directly inhibits the activation of macrophages and the release of cytokines at the site of injury. It serves to localize invasive events from several local sites, mobilizes defenses, and creates memory to improve chances for survival. At the same time it prevents spillage of inflammatory products into the circulation.

When the threat is gone, these systems must be shut off. In the setting of repeated hits from multiple stressors, lack of adaptation with repeated exposure, a delayed shutdown, or an inadequate response that leads to compensatory hyperactivity of other mediators (eg, impaired counter-regulation of cytokines [inflammatory state] caused by inadequate secretion of glucocorticoids) results in wear and tear from chronic overactivity or underactivity of these allostatic systems (allostatic load).

Insulin resistance

The most accepted and unifying hypothesis to describe the pathophysiology of the metabolic syndrome is insulin resistance, although quantification of insulin action in vivo is not always strongly related to the presence of the syndrome [26]. Alterations that are not included in the diagnostic criteria for the metabolic syndrome but have been reported in association with insulin resistance are depicted in Box 1. Several studies have reported an association between insulin resistance and depressive disorder, although the association is not seen universally [27–30].

Insulin resistance and major depression share several disturbances in the aforementioned physiologic systems that include the HPA axis, the autonomic nervous system, the immune system, platelets, and endothelial function.

Activation of the hypothalamus-pituitary-adrenal axis

Depression is often accompanied by hypercortisolemia. Associated findings include attenuation of the corticotropin response to the administration of corticotrophin-releasing factor and nonsuppression of cortisol secretion after dexamethasone administration. Hypercortisolemia in association with blunted growth and sex hormones promotes central obesity and contributes to increased insulin resistance and diabetes among depressed subjects [31]. The presence of hypercortisolemia in insulin resistance has been documented in some, but not all, studies. A small case-control study has shown some evidence for increased cortisol production in the metabolic syndrome as well [32]. Notably, a contributory role for cortisol metabolism in the pathogenesis of the metabolic syndrome has been postulated. Deregulation of 11 betahydroxysteroiddehydrogenase, an enzyme that converts cortisol into cortisone (which cannot activate the glucocorticoid receptor), may result in excess cortisol exposure at the tissue level and induce visceral adiposity [33].

Autonomic nervous system imbalance

In healthy persons the autonomic balance in the body varies depending on the activity it performs. The sympathetic nervous system is predominant in the active ("fight, fright, and flight") period, whereas the parasympathetic nervous system rules the body in the inactive ("rest and digest") period. With physical activity in the active period, the movement apparatus requires blood, and the digestive apparatus slows down; the opposite holds for the inactive period. Thus, blood vessels in these different regions must receive different autonomic signals depending on the time of the day. Recently, neuroanatomic studies have shown the existence of compartmentalization of autonomic motor neurons, thus providing a basis for selective changes of the sympatho-parasympathetic balance in different compartments of the body [34]. Parasympathetic input to fat tissue has been shown to enhance insulin sensitivity and fat accumulation.

Abnormalities in autonomic nervous system activity are consistent findings in depression, insulin resistance, and, more recently, the metabolic syndrome. Impaired autonomic function previously has been associated with elevated concentrations of serum insulin and decreased insulin sensitivity (markers of insulin resistance), independent of glucose levels [35,36]. Depressed patients commonly manifest higher resting heart rates than healthy controls and exhibit autonomic nervous system dysfunction, including diminished heart rate variability (HRV), baroreflex dysfunction, and increased QT variability, all of which have been linked to increased cardiac mortality, including sudden death [37].

Decreased HRV seems to be predictive of diabetes. HRV reflects fluctuations in autonomic inputs to the heart and comprises both parasympathetic and sympathetic inputs. In the Atherosclerosis Risk in Communities study, subjects who had reduced HRV in the low-frequency (LF) range (a marker of decreased parasympathetic input) and high resting heart rate (a global marker of poor autonomic nervous system modulation) were at increased risk for developing type 2 diabetes, and low levels of physical activity and central adiposity played a large role in this association [38]. Persons who have low HRV and correspondingly low LF power presumably have considerable resting sympathetic input. Increased sympathetic activation leads to enhanced catecholamine release and consequent increases in circulating free fatty acids and thus increased insulin resistance.

It has been postulated that in the metabolic syndrome the sympathetic branch prevails in the thorax (heart and large vessels) and movement compartment (skeletal muscles), leading to high blood pressure and impaired glucose uptake by the muscle (ie, insulin resistance). In the intra-abdominal compartment, however, the autonomic nervous system balance is shifted in favor of the parasympathetic branch, resulting in increased insulin secretion and growth of intra-abdominal fat tissue [34]. Cardiac sympathetic predominance and increased catecholamine output has recently been shown in subjects who have metabolic syndrome [32]. Notably, psychosocial factors seemed to explain a considerable part of this association.

Endothelial dysfunction

The endothelium is a critical determinant of vascular tone, reactivity, inflammation, vascular remodeling, maintenance of vascular patency, and blood fluidity. In the healthy state the normal homeostatic properties of the endothelium favors vasodilatation, low permeability, anticoagulation, and poor adhesiveness with respect to leukocytes and platelets. Different forms of injury (eg, hyperlipidemia, diabetes, hypertension, and smoking) increase the vasomotor tone and the vasomotor response of arteries to various stimuli, including mental stress, increase the adhesiveness and permeability of the endothelium, and induce a procoagulant state as a result of the formation of vasoactive molecules, cytokines, and growth factors. The concomitant and ongoing inflammatory response at the tissue as well as systemic level supposedly propagates tissue injury and results in progressive atherosclerosis [39].

Depression is associated with a heightened incidence of endothelial dysfunction (ie, impaired flow-mediated vasodilation) among various cohorts, including young and otherwise healthy depressed patients [40]. Impaired endothelial function is a putative mechanism that links insulin resistance and cardiovascular disease, including hypertension [41–43]. It comes as no surprise that endothelial function is found to be impaired in the metabolic syndrome as well [44].

Thus far, the putative mechanisms behind the association between endothelial dysfunction and depression are largely unknown but may involve stimulation of the HPA axis, activation of the sympathetic nervous system, endothelial dysfunction, and also potential synergy induced by peripheral effects. One such mechanism in the presence of the metabolic syndrome has recently been postulated as vasocrine signaling from perivascular fat that inhibits insulin-mediated capillary recruitment through the release of the adipocytokine tumor necrosis factor [45].

Platelets

Insulin resistance is associated with changes in platelets (and fibrinolysis and coagulation) that favor a prothrombotic state [46]. Depressed patients also may develop significant impairments in platelet function. In the presence of concomitant risk factors for coronary artery disease, enhanced platelet reactivity and release of platelet products such as platelet factor 4 and b-thromboglobulin, increased concentration of functional glycoprotein IIb/IIIa receptors, and a hyperactive 5-hydroxytryptamine transporter2A receptor signal transduction system and related increased responsiveness of platelets to serotonin have been shown [47]. Whatever its cause, enhanced platelet reactivity may contribute to cardiovascular complications in the setting of atherosclerotic disease. For this reason a cardioprotective effect of selective serotonin reuptake inhibitors has been postulated but remains to be proven [48].

Inflammation

Lately, much attention has been directed to inflammation as the central feature of atherosclerosis. The balance between inflammatory and anti-inflammatory activity in the vessel wall governs the progression of atherosclerosis, in close interactions with various metabolic factors of which lipid and products of lipid peroxidation are the most prominent [49]. Activated immune cells in the atherosclerotic plaque produce inflammatory cytokines (interferon-gamma, interleukin-1, and tumor necrosis factor) that induce the production of substantial amounts of interleukin-6. When these cytokines spill into the systemic circulation, interleukin-6 stimulates the production of large amounts of acute-phase reactants, including C-reactive protein, serum amyloid A, and fibrinogen, especially in the liver. The inflammatory process in the atherosclerotic artery thus may lead to increased blood levels of inflammatory cytokines and other acute-phase reactants. A moderately elevated C-reactive protein level on a highly sensitive immunoassay has been shown to be an independent risk factor for coronary artery disease in a healthy population [43]. Levels of C-reactive protein and interleukin-6 are elevated in patients who have unstable angina and myocardial infarction, with higher levels predicting worse prognosis [50]. Visceral adipose tissue has turned out to be another major production site of these cytokines and thus may contribute to this inflammatory burden in persons who have the metabolic syndrome.

Depression has also been found to be associated with increases in C-re-active protein, interleukin-6, tumor necrosis factor, and other inflammatory proteins [51,52]. The possibility of insufficient dampening of the inflammatory response related to diminished glucocorticoid sensitivity in depression has been suggested [52]. Whether this reduced sensitivity relates to increased cardiovascular risk has yet not been studied.

The significance of psychosocial stress

It follows from the previous sections that psychosocial factors, such as a physical threat, may induce an allostatic response and thus have profound effects on the integrity of the body and add to the wear and tear on tissues and organs. Excessive weight gain, for example, is a physical threat that, in turn, may be the outcome of a complex interaction between an adverse life style caused by psychosocial factors in the setting of a genetic predisposition to metabolic inflexibility [53] and complex cross-talk between the brain and the gut. In this section, the effect of psychosocial factors on the cardiovascular system and some new insight on the relationship between psychosocial factors and food intake are addressed.

Wear and tear on the cardiovascular system

Semiacute psychosocial stress is associated with increased cardiovascular morbidity and mortality. The incidence of sudden death increases directly after a major disaster [54]. Also, reversible cardiac failure caused by sudden emotional distress has been reported [55]. A major role in the pathogenesis of these complications has been ascribed to activation of the HPA axis. Evidence of neurohumoral arousal and elevation of arterial blood pressure has been noted in situations associated with acute and subacute stress [56,57]. Exaggerated physiologic responses to acute stressors also have been shown in depressed, hostile, and low-SES subjects [37,58,59]. Chronic stress and hostility have been linked to increased reactivity of the fibrinogen system and of platelets, both of which increase the risk of myocardial infarction [60,61]. Also, tension and anxiety over a more prolonged period of time have been observed to be independent risk factors of incident coronary heart disease, atrial fibrillation, and mortality [62]. This notion is corroborated by animal studies among Cynomolgus monkeys that have reported an association between social isolation and hypercortisolemia and reversible increases in resting heart rates, suggesting that social factors promote atherogenesis through activation of the HPA axis and the autonomic nervous system [63,64].

Recently, the increased mortality of elderly people in the year following the hospital admittance of a spouse has been demonstrated [65]. Notably, the hospitalization of a spouse was associated with a risk of death for the partner within the first 30 days that was almost as great as the risk associated with the death of a spouse. Although factors related to harmful behavior by the partner who has been left behind cannot be ruled out in the latter study, the time frame is such that a direct stress-mediated effect is suggested.

Other studies have linked sympathetic hyperresponsivity to the induction of myocardial ischemia during exercise and mental stress and to predictions of the future development of hypertension and progression of atherosclerosis [66–72]. Increased systemic vascular resistance during mental stress testing is the most significant hemodynamic factor associated with mental stress–induced myocardial ischemia and most likely is the result of peripheral endothelial dysfunction [73]. Inhibition of cortisol production has been shown to prevent mental stress–induced endothelial dysfunction and baroreflex impairment, again pointing to a significant role of the HPA axis [74]. Interestingly, endothelial dysfunction after mental stress has been shown in hypertensive subjects but not in patients who have hypercholesterolemia [75]. This finding is noteworthy because both hypertension and hypercholesterolemia are risk factors for atherosclerosis and cardiovascular disease, and endothelial dysfunction is a distinct feature of both diseases. These findings suggest different underlying mechanisms for endothelial dysfunction to account for the observed difference. When a similar stressor exerts a distinct response in subjects that, depending on the disease, that makes them more susceptible to atherosclerosis, the question is raised whether different stressors might likewise evoke different pathophysiologic mechanisms and, possibly, different atherosclerotic manifestations. The latter possibility is supported by animal data. Exposure of Watanabe heritable hyperlipidemic rabbits to two different chronic stressors (ie, an unstable social environment or social isolation) resulted in more atherosclerosis than seen in a control group, but the two stressed groups exhibited different metabolic consequences and patterns of accrued atherosclerosis [76]. Animals that were socially isolated were relatively sedentary, gained more body weight, and developed more profound hyperinsulinemia than the socially unstable group. They exhibited no stressful behaviors, such as cowering, vocalizations, or sleep or feeding disturbances, and had low corticosterone levels compared with the socially unstable group. At the same time they had higher resting heart rates and more pronounced abdominal aortic atherosclerosis.

The extent to which psychosocial factors affect the cardiovascular system through its interaction with the immune system has not been widely investigated thus far, but its potential significance is suggested by studies that have documented increased severity of the common cold related to psychologic stress and lack of social support [77,78]. As in depression, insufficient dampening of the inflammatory response related to diminished glucocorticoid sensitivity might be of importance [52]. Whether facilitation of sustained expression of inflammatory mediators under the influence of psychosocial factors might foster cardiovascular complications remains speculative.

Food, stress, and reward

The limbic system is a complex set of structures that includes the hypothalamus, the hippocampus, the amygdala, and several nearby areas. It seems to be primarily responsible for emotional life and the formation of memories. As described earlier, the hypothalamus is mainly responsible for homeostasis and thereby regulates heart rate, blood pressure, breathing, and gastrointestinal motility and also regulates behavior and arousal in response to hunger, thirst, and emotional circumstances (eg, pain, pleasure, sex, fear, or hostility).

Repeated stress especially affects the hippocampus, which participates in verbal memory and is particularly important for the memory of context, that is, the time and place of events that have a strong emotional bias [23]. Moreover, glucocorticoids are involved in remembering the context in which an emotionally laden event took place. The hippocampus also regulates the stress response and acts to inhibit the response of the HPA axis to stress.

The hypothalamus, especially the arcuate nucleus, is relatively accessible to circulating factors and receives inputs from other areas of the brain, including the tractus solitarius and the area postrema [79]. The hypothalamus receives signals that relate to total energy stores in fat and to immediate changes in energy availability, including insulin, leptin, and nutrients within the gut. Afferent signals from the gut to the brain are carried in vagal and splanchnic nerve pathways. The gut also releases several hormones that have incretin- (GLP-1, GIP), hunger- (Ghrelin), and satiety-stimulating (PYY, GLP-1, OXM) actions [79]. In addition, major afferent input originates from the adipose tissue. The adipocyte is now recognized as a bona fide endocrine cell. Adipocyte hormones such as adiponectin, resistin, and visfatin influence appetite, glucose homeostasis and insulin sensitivity, and vascular function, among other functions [80].

The hypothalamus integrates these peripheral and central signals and exerts homeostatic control over food intake, levels of physical activity, basal energy expenditure, and endocrine systems.

There is no doubt that food intake in humans is influenced by emotional factors, social cues, and learned behavior. Functional neuroimaging techniques have provided the first insight in the response of the brain to nutritional stimuli. Differences regarding both the need to eat and the pleasure of eating between obese and lean individuals have been noted [81].

In obese individuals the decrease in hypothalamic activity following a meal is significantly reduced compared with lean individuals. Importantly, the neural substrates of the sensory perception of food overlap extensively with the brain representation of reward. Dopamine is the neurotransmitter that plays a central role in mediating the anticipation of reward. Abnormalities in dopaminergic transmission can be evidenced in obese individuals [82]. A decreased D2 receptor function in this same reward area of the brain has been shown, varying inversely with body mass index.

Various other data suggest that the link between chronic psychologic distress and adverse behavior such as overeating may be centrally mediated [83,84]. Normally, glucocorticoids help end acute stress responses by exerting negative feedback on the HPA axis. In contrast, it has been shown in a rat model that glucocorticoids occupy central glucocorticoid receptors during chronic stress, with resultant activation of the chronic stress response network, including continued glucocorticoid production [85]. This combination of chronic stress and high glucocorticoid levels seems to stimulate a preferential desire to ingest sweet and fatty foods, presumably by affecting dopaminergic transmission in areas of the brain associated with motivation and reward [86]. Similar to observations in obese individuals, diminished dopamine D2–binding potential within midbrain systems under conditions of chronic stress has been shown by positron-emission tomography scanning in the Cynomolgus monkey [87]. It has been demonstrated that in humans this area is involved specifically in food motivation [88].

Recent evidence also links brain areas associated with reward with those that sense physical pain. It is common notion that chronic pain can cause depression, and depression can increase pain. Most patients who have depression also present with mainly physical symptoms [89]. Studies using functional MRI have shown that social rejection lights up brain areas that are also key regions in the response to physical pain. The area of the anterior cingulate cortex that is activated by visceral pain also is activated in cases of social rejection [90]. The importance of these brain areas is underscored by the observation that the right ventral prefrontal cortex that mitigates emotional distress caused by pain is activated when placebo administration relieves pain [91].

These stress-induced changes (ie, allostatic load) are not without consequences. MRI has shown that stress-related disorders such as recurrent depressive illness or posttraumatic stress disorder are associated with atrophy of the hippocampus [92,93]. Impairment of the hippocampus decreases the reliability and accuracy of contextual memories. This decrement may exacerbate stress by preventing access to the information needed to decide that a situation is not an emotional or physical threat. Also, the suppression of routine sensory input from the body that normally occurs might, under these circumstances, be felt as discomfort or pain. There is evidence that antidepressants can reverse these changes [94].

Integrative approach to treatment

From the previous discussion, it has become clear that some parts of the pathophysiologic basis for the association between depression, cardiovascular diseases, and the metabolic syndrome are gradually becoming clearer, but these associations are complex and should be modeled over the lifetime. Because exposure to various disease risks (ie, physical, psychosocial stress,

and behavioral stressors) in humans changes over time, and risks cluster together in variable fashion, it is evident that a simple cause-and-effect approach does not fit the individual patient. One must define the chain of
risk (as discussed later) with its mediating and modifying factors that
have played and still play a role. For this reason an integrated approach
with close attention to the history and actual needs and expectations of
the individual patient in both the biologic and psychosocial domains is
necessary.

It is not necessary to identify with certainty or to address every component
cause or risk to prevent or avoid further deterioration of a disease. To understand this notion, one needs to address the issue of causation once more.
When one defines a cause of a disease as an event, condition, or characteristic
that preceded the disease and without which the disease either would not have
occurred at all or would not have occurred until some later time, it follows
that no specific event, condition, or characteristic is sufficient by itself to produce disease [95]. A sufficient cause can be defined as a set of minimal conditions and events that over time inevitably produce disease. A minimal cause
implies that all of the conditions or events are necessary for disease occurrence. For a disease to occur, a multitude of component causes are needed
that act over time in a chain of risk that in turn involves mediating and modifying factors. The importance of this notion is that most identified causes are
neither necessary nor sufficient to produce disease. Vice-versa, a cause need
not be either necessary or sufficient for its removal to result in disease prevention in some individuals. Because each individual has a unique chain of risks
over time, it should come as no surprise that until now it has been difficult to
prove that treatment for depression benefits the cardiovascular outcome after
myocardial infarction [96].

This lack of proof, however, does not preclude the possibility that some
subjects do benefit in this respect. Although the therapeutic advice in this
context should be based on the overall outcome of such intervention studies,

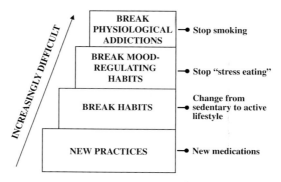

Fig. 2. Hierarchy of interventions relative to their complexity. (*From* Rozanski A. Integrating
psychologic approaches into the behavioral management of cardiac patents. Psychosom Med
2005;67(Suppl 1):S68; with permission.)

it is important to pay proper attention to all three biopsychosocial domains, and thus the individual situation of a patient, and to act as one deems necessary for the general health of the patient. This approach is, at the same time, the most difficult, because inducing patients to make behavioral changes is much more difficult than prescribing some medication (Fig. 2) [97]. Such an approach, however, will best address the patients' physical, emotional, and social well being and, importantly, create a trusting patient–doctor relationship. It is evident that current medical services, which by definition act upon simple cause-and-effect disease models, do not suffice to provide this kind of patient-tailored therapy.

References

[1] Eckel RH, Grundy SM, Zimmet PZ. The metabolic syndrome. Lancet 2005;365:1415–28.
[2] Alberti KG, Zimmet P, Shaw J, for the IDF Epidemiology Task Force Consensus Group. The metabolic syndrome—a new worldwide definition. Lancet 2005;366:1059–62.
[3] Kahn R, Buse J, Ferrannini E, et al. The American Diabetes Association. European Association for the Study of Diabetes. The metabolic syndrome: time for a critical appraisal: joint statement from the American Diabetes Association and the European Association for the Study of Diabetes. Diabetes Care 2005;28:2289–304.
[4] Knowler WC, Barrett-Connor E, Fowler SE, et al. Diabetes Prevention Program Research Group. Reduction in the incidence of type 2 diabetes with lifestyle intervention or metformin. N Engl J Med 2002;346:393–403.
[5] Engum A, Mykletun A, Midthjell K, et al. Depression and diabetes: a large population-based study of sociodemographic, lifestyle, and clinical factors associated with depression in type 1 and type 2 diabetes. Diabetes Care 2005;28:1904–9.
[6] Kinder LS, Carnethon MR, Palaniappan LP, et al. Depression and the metabolic syndrome in young adults: findings from the Third National Health and Nutrition Examination Survey. Psychosom Med 2004;66:316–22.
[7] Haslam DW, James WP. Obesity. Lancet 2005;366:1197–209.
[8] Everson-Rose SA, Meyer PM, Powell LH, et al. Depressive symptoms, insulin resistance, and risk of diabetes in women at midlife. Diabetes Care 2004;27:2856–62.
[9] Rugulies R. Depression as a predictor for coronary heart disease. A review and meta-analysis. Am J Prev Med 2002;23(1):51–61.
[10] Rozanski A, Blumenthal JA, Davidson KW, et al. The epidemiology, pathophysiology, and management of psychosocial risk factors in cardiac practice: the emerging field of behavioral cardiology. J Am Coll Cardiol 2005;45:637–51.
[11] Yusuf S, Hawken S, Ounpuu S, et al. INTERHEART Study Investigators. Effect of potentially modifiable risk factors associated with myocardial infarction in 52 countries (the INTERHEART study): case-control study. Lancet 2004;364:937–52.
[12] Alexopoulos GS, Meyers BS, Young RC, et al. 'Vascular depression' hypothesis. Arch Gen Psychiatry 1997;54:915–22.
[13] Ben-Shlomo Y, Kuh D. A life course approach to chronic disease epidemiology: conceptual models, empirical challenges and interdisciplinary perspectives. Int J Epidemiol 2002;31: 285–93.
[14] Frankel S, Elwood P, Sweetnam P, et al. Birthweight, body-mass index in middle age, and incident coronary heart disease. Lancet 1996;348:1478–80.
[15] Lithell HO, McKeigue PM, Berglund L, et al. Relation of size at birth to non-insulin dependent diabetes and insulin concentrations in men aged 50–60 years. BMJ 1996;312:406–10.
[16] Eriksson JG, Forsen T, Tuomilehto J, et al. Early growth and coronary heart disease in later life: longitudinal study. BMJ 2001;322:949–53.

[17] Wiles NJ, Peters TJ, Leon DA, et al. Birth weight and psychological distress at age 45–51 years: results from the Aberdeen Children of the 1950s cohort study. Br J Psychiatry 2005; 187:21–8.

[18] Kuh D, Hardy R, Langenberg C, et al. Mortality in adults aged 26–54 years related to socio-economic conditions in childhood and adulthood: post war birth cohort study. BMJ 2002; 325:1076–80.

[19] Kaplan GA. Going back to understand the future: socioeconomic position and survival after myocardial infarction. Ann Intern Med 2006;144:137–9

[20] Brunner EJ, Marmot MG, Nanchahal K, et al. Social inequality in coronary risk: central obesity and the metabolic syndrome. Evidence from the Whitehall II study. Diabetologia 1997;40(11):1341–9.

[21] Fryers T, Melzer D, Jenkins R, et al. The distribution of the common mental disorders: social inequalities in Europe. Clin Pract Epidemol Ment Health 2005;1:14.

[22] Selye H. Syndrome produced by diverse nocuous agents. Nature 1936;138:32.

[23] McEwen BS. Protective and damaging effects of stress mediators. N Engl J Med 1998;338(3): 171–9.

[24] Craig AD. How do you feel? Interoception: the sense of the physiological condition of the body. Nat Rev Neurosci 2002;3:655–66.

[25] Tracey KJ. The inflammatory reflex. Nature 2002;420(6917):853–9.

[26] Hanley AJ, Wagenknecht LE, D'Agostino RB Jr, et al. Identification of subjects with insulin resistance and beta-cell dysfunction using alternative definitions of the metabolic syndrome. Diabetes 2003;52(11):2740–7.

[27] Okamura F, Tashiro A, Utumi A, et al. Insulin resistance in patients with depression and its changes during the clinical course of depression: minimal model analysis. Metabolism 2000; 49:1255–60.

[28] Ramasubbu R. Insulin resistance: a metabolic link between depressive disorder and athero-sclerotic vascular diseases. Med Hypotheses 2002;59:537–51.

[29] Lawlor DA, Smith GD, Ebrahim S. British Women's Heart and Health Study. Association of insulin resistance with depression: cross sectional findings from the British Women's Heart and Health Study. BMJ 2003;327:1383–4.

[30] Timonen M, Laakso M, Jokelainen J, et al. Insulin resistance and depression: cross sectional study. BMJ 2005;330:17–8.

[31] Weber-Hamann B, Hentschel F, Kniest A, et al. Hypercortisolemic depression is associated with increased intra-abdominal fat. Psychosom Med 2002;64:274–7.

[32] Brunner EJ, Hemingway H, Walker BR, et al. Adrenocortical, autonomic, and inflamma-tory causes of the metabolic syndrome: nested case-control study. Circulation 2002;106: 2659–65.

[33] Bujalska IJ, Kumar S, Stewart PM. Does central obesity reflect "Cushing's disease of the omentum"? Lancet 1997;349:1210–3.

[34] Kreier F, Yilmaz A, Kalsbeek A, et al. Hypothesis: shifting the equilibrium from activity to food leads to autonomic unbalance and the metabolic syndrome. Diabetes 2003;52:2652–6.

[35] Festa A, D'Agostino R Jr, Hales CN, et al. Heart rate in relation to insulin sensitivity and insulin secretion in nondiabetic subjects. Diabetes Care 2000;23:624–8.

[36] Panzer C, Lauer MS, Brieke A, et al. Association of fasting plasma glucose with heart rate recovery in healthy adults: a population-based study. Diabetes 2002;51:803–7.

[37] Carney RM, Freedland KE, Veith RC. Depression, the autonomic nervous system, and cor-onary heart disease. Psychosom Med 2005;67(Suppl 1):S29–33.

[38] Carnethon MR, Golden SH, Folsom AR, et al. Prospective investigation of autonomic ner-vous system function and the development of type 2 diabetes: the Atherosclerosis Risk In Communities study, 1987–1998. Circulation 2003;107:2190–5.

[39] Ross R. Atherosclerosis—an inflammatory disease. N Engl J Med 1999;340:115–26.

[40] Rajagopalan S, Brook R, Rubenfire M, et al. Abnormal brachial artery flow-mediated vaso-dilation in young adults with major depression. Am J Cardiol 2001;88:196–8.

[41] Vitale Despres JP, Lamarche B, Mauriege P, et al. Hyperinsulinemia as an independent risk factor for ischemic heart disease. N Engl J Med 1996;334(15):952–7.

[42] Serne EH, Gans RO, ter Maaten JC, et al. Capillary recruitment is impaired in essential hypertension and relates to insulin's metabolic and vascular actions. Cardiovasc Res 2001; 49(1):161–8.

[43] Vita JA, Keaney JF Jr, Larson MG, et al. Brachial artery vasodilator function and systemic inflammation in the Framingham Offspring Study. Circulation 2004;110:3604–9.

[44] Vitale C, Mercuro G, Cornoldi A, et al. Metformin improves endothelial function in patients with metabolic syndrome. J Intern Med 2005;258(3):250–6.

[45] Yudkin JS, Eringa E, Stehouwer CD. "Vasocrine" signalling from perivascular fat: a mechanism linking insulin resistance to vascular disease. Lancet 2005;365(9473):1817–20.

[46] Schneider DJ. Abnormalities of coagulation, platelet function, and fibrinolysis associated with syndromes of insulin resistance. Coron Artery Dis 2005;16(8):473–6.

[47] Bruce EC, Musselman DL. Depression, alterations in platelet function, and ischemic heart disease. Psychosom Med 2005;67(Suppl 1):S34–6.

[48] Taylor CB, Youngblood ME, Catellier D, et al. Effects of antidepressant medication on morbidity and mortality in depressed patients after myocardial infarction. Arch Gen Psychiatry 2005;62(7):792–8.

[49] Hansson GK. Inflammation, atherosclerosis, and coronary artery disease. N Engl J Med 2005;352:1685–95.

[50] Danesh J, Wheeler JG, Hirschfield GM, et al. C-reactive protein and other circulating markers of inflammation in the prediction of coronary heart disease. N Engl J Med 2004; 350:1387–97.

[51] Anisman H, Merali Z. Cytokines, stress, and depressive illness. Brain Behav Immun 2002;16: 513–24.

[52] Miller GE, Rohleder N, Stetler C, et al. Clinical depression and regulation of the inflammatory response during acute stress. Psychosom Med 2005;67(5):679–87.

[53] Kelley DE, Mandarino LJ. Fuel selection in human skeletal muscle in insulin resistance: a reexamination. Diabetes 2000;49(5):677–83.

[54] Leor J, Poole WK, Kloner RA. Sudden cardiac death triggered by an earthquake. N Engl J Med 1996;334:413–9.

[55] Wittstein IS, Thiemann DR, Lima JA, et al. Neurohumoral features of myocardial stunning due to sudden emotional stress. N Engl J Med 2005;352:539–48.

[56] Schnall PL, Pieper C, Schwartz JE, et al. The relationship between job strain, work place diastolic blood pressure, and left ventricular mass index. JAMA 1990;263:1929–35.

[57] Theorell T, Perski A, Akerstedt T, et al. Changes in job strain in relation to changes in physiological state. A longitudinal study. Scand J Work Environ Health 1988;14(3):189–96.

[58] Suarez EC, Kuhn CM, Schanberg SM, et al. Neuroendocrine, cardiovascular, and emotional responses of hostile men: the role of interpersonal challenge. Psychosom Med 1998;60:78–88.

[59] Rosmond R, Bjorntorp P. Occupational status, cortisol secretory pattern, and visceral obesity in middle-aged men. Obes Res 2000;8:445–50.

[60] Raikkonen K, Lassila R, Keltikangas-Jarvinen L, et al. Association of chronic stress with plasminogen activator inhibitor-1 in healthy middle-aged men. Arterioscler Thromb Vasc Biol 1996;16:363–7.

[61] Markowe HLJ, Marmot MG, Shipley MJ, et al. Fibrinogen: a possible link between social class and coronary heart disease. BMJ 1985;291:1312–4.

[62] Eaker ED, Sullivan LM, Kelly-Hayes M, et al. Tension and anxiety and the prediction of the 10-year incidence of coronary heart disease, atrial fibrillation, and total mortality: the Framingham Offspring study. Psychosom Med 2005;67:692–6.

[63] Sapolsky RM, Alberts SC, Altman J. Hypercortisolism associated with social subordinance or social isolation among wild baboons. Arch Gen Psychiatry 1997;54:1137–43.

[64] Watson SL, Shively CA, Kaplan JR, et al. Effects of chronic social separation on cardiovascular disease risk factors in female Cynomolgus monkeys. Atherosclerosis 1998;137:259–66.

[65] Christakis NA, Allison PD. Mortality after the hospitalization of a spouse. N Engl J Med 2006;354:719–30.

[66] Kral BG, Becker LC, Blumenthal RS, et al. Exaggerated reactivity to mental stress is associated with exercise-induced myocardial ischemia in an asymptomatic high-risk population. Circulation 1997;96:4246–53.

[67] Krantz DS, Helmers KF, Bairey CN, et al. Cardiovascular reactivity and mental stress-induced myocardial ischemia in patients with coronary artery disease. Psychosom Med 1991;53:1–12.

[68] Matthews KA, Woodall KL, Allen MT. Cardiovascular reactivity to stress predicts future blood pressure status. Hypertension 1993;22:479–85.

[69] Everson SA, Kaplan GA, Goldberg DE, et al. Anticipatory blood pressure response to exercise predicts future high blood pressure in middle-aged men. Hypertension 1996;27: 1059–64.

[70] Everson SA, Lynch JW, Chesney MA, et al. Interaction of workplace demands and cardiovascular reactivity in progression of carotid atherosclerosis: population based study. BMJ 1997;314:553–8.

[71] Kamarck TW, Everson SA, Kaplan GA, et al. Exaggerated blood pressure responses during mental stress are associated with enhanced carotid atherosclerosis in middle-aged Finnish men: findings from the Kuopio Ischemic Heart Disease Study. Circulation 1997;96:3842–8.

[72] Matthews KA, Owens JF, Kuller LH, et al. Stress induced pulse pressure change predicts women's carotid atherosclerosis. Stroke 1998;29:1525–30.

[73] Spieker LE, Hurlimann D, Ruschitzka F, et al. Mental stress induces prolonged endothelial dysfunction via endothelin-A receptors. Circulation 2002;105(24):2817–20.

[74] Broadley AJ, Korszun A, Abdelaal E, et al. Inhibition of cortisol production with metyrapone prevents mental stress-induced endothelial dysfunction and baroreflex impairment. J Am Coll Cardiol 2005;46(2):344–50.

[75] Cardillo C, Kilcoyne CM, Cannon RO III, et al. Impairment of the nitric oxide-mediated vasodilator response to mental stress in hypertensive but not in hypercholesterolemic patients. J Am Coll Cardiol 1998;32(5):1207–13.

[76] McCabe PM, Gonzales JA, Zaias J, et al. Social environment influences the progression of atherosclerosis in the Watanabe heritable hyperlipidemic rabbit. Circulation 2002;105: 354–9.

[77] Cohen S, Tyrrell DAJ, Smith AP. Psychological stress and susceptibility to the common cold. N Engl J Med 1991;325:606–12.

[78] Cohen S, Doyle WJ, Skoner DP, et al. Social ties and susceptibility to the common cold. JAMA 1997;277(24):1940–4.

[79] Badman MK, Flier JS. The gut and energy balance: visceral allies in the obesity wars. Science 2005;307(5717):1909–14.

[80] Kershaw EE, Flier JS. Adipose tissue as an endocrine organ. J Clin Endocrinol Metab 2004; 89(6):2548–56.

[81] Tataranni PA, DelParigi A. Functional neuroimaging: a new generation of human brain studies in obesity research. Obes Rev 2003;4(4):229–38.

[82] Wang GJ, Volkow ND, Logan J, et al. Brain dopamine and obesity. Lancet 2001;357:354–7.

[83] McElroy SL, Kotwal R, Malhotra S, et al. Are mood disorders and obesity related? A review for the mental health professional. J Clin Psychiatry 2004;65:634–51.

[84] Dallman MF, La Fluer S, Pecoraro NC, et al. Minireview: glucocorticoids—food intake, abdominal obesity, and wealthy nations in 2004. Endocrinology 2004;145:2633–8.

[85] Bhatnagar S, Dallman M. Neuroanatomical basis for facilitation of hypothalamic-pituitary-adrenal responses to a novel stressor after chronic stress. Neuroscience 1998;84:1025–39.

[86] Lindley SE, Bengoechea TG, Schatzberg AF, et al. Glucocorticoid effects on mesotelencephalic dopamine neurotransmission. Neuropsychopharmacology 1999;21:399–407.

[87] Morgan D, Grant KA, Gage HD, et al. Social dominance in monkeys: dopamine D2 receptors and cocaine self-administration. Nat Neurosci 2002;5:169–74.

[88] Volkow ND, Wang GJ, Fowler JS, et al. "Nonhedonic" food motivation in humans involves dopamine in the dorsal striatum and methylphenidate amplifies this effect. Synapse 2002;44: 175–80.
[89] Kirmayer LJ, Robbins JM, Dworkind M, et al. Somatization and the recognition of depression and anxiety in primary care. Am J Psychiatry 1993;150(5):734–41.
[90] Eisenberger NI, Lieberman MD, Williams KD. Does rejection hurt? An FMRI study of social exclusion. Science 2003;302(5643):290–2.
[91] Wager TD, Rilling JK, Smith EE, et al. Placebo-induced changes in FMRI in the anticipation and experience of pain. Science 2004;303(5661):1162–7.
[92] Sapolsky RM. Why stress is bad for your brain. Science 1996;273:749–50.
[93] McEwen BS, Magarinos AM. Stress effects on morphology and function of the hippocampus. Ann N Y Acad Sci 1997;821:271–84.
[94] Ebmeier KP, Donaghey C, Steele JD. Recent developments and current controversies in depression. Lancet 2006;367(9505):153–67.
[95] Rothman KJ, Greenland S. Causation and causal inference in epidemiology. Am J Public Health 2005;95(Suppl 1):S144–50.
[96] Rees K, Bennett P, West R, et al. Psychological interventions for coronary heart disease. Cochrane Database Syst Rev 2004;4:CD002902.
[97] Rozanski A. Integrating psychologic approaches into the behavioral management of cardiac patients. Psychosom Med 2005;67(Suppl 1):S67–73.

ELSEVIER
SAUNDERS

Med Clin N Am 90 (2006) 593–601

THE MEDICAL
CLINICS
OF NORTH AMERICA

Vulnerability in the Elderly: Frailty

Joris P.J. Slaets, MD, PhD

Department of Internal Medicine, University Medical Center Groningen,
Hanzeplein 1, 9700 RB, Groningen, The Netherlands

Earlier in this issue the highly complex interrelations between the multitude of factors that are active in the pathophysiology of the metabolic syndrome were described. Based on that an argument was made for an integrated approach, even though the current available research does not support such an approach to its full extent. From the patient's perspective, however, it seems more than justified to go for such an approach [1]. This article builds on this perspective and further elaborates on it in a specific, but highly important, population—the frail elderly. Patients, who suffer by definition from several diseases or functional limitations of organ systems that interact, need integrated assessment and care for these reasons.

The concepts

It is acknowledged widely that different multifactorial diseases share the same risk factors, both genetic and environmental. Second, multifactorial diseases cluster (ie, patients with one such disease are more likely to develop additional diseases). Multifactorial diseases are the result of multiple risk factors. Examples are depression, cancer, chronic obstructive pulmonary disease, and cardiovascular and endocrine diseases; together they make up the most common disorders in adulthood, and are responsible for the use of most health care resources. So, most complex patients have different multifactorial diseases. Most factors that are associated with multifactorial diseases are the result of an interaction between genetic and environmental risk factors. Complex risk factors are the result of interactions between multiple genetic or environmental factors. Examples are body weight, personality traits, social support, epigenetic factors, and plasma cortisol level. Usually these associations are not understood completely, but their roles as risk factors have been established (eg, by proven benefit from intervention on such a risk factor). The understanding of comorbidity and multifactorial risk

E-mail address: j.p.j.slaets@int.umcg.nl

factors is important for the treatment of complex patients. Dealing with all of the interacting and adaptive systems makes health care more complex with less degrees of certainty [2].

Frailty and age

The general concept of vulnerability has a specific meaning in the context of the elderly. Frailty can be seen as increasing vulnerability associated with aging. According to Verbrugge [3], frailty can be seen as a syndrome in which more areas of functioning decline with aging. In this way frailty is a precursor state of functional limitations and disability associated with the aging process itself; the comorbidity of chronic diseases; and multiple risk factors, including psychosocial and functional limitations.

The formal definition of comorbidity is the concurrent presence of two or more medically diagnosed diseases in the same individual. With aging, comorbidity increases markedly, in large part because the frequency of individual chronic conditions increases with age. As a result, at ages 65 to 79 years 35.3% of the population in the United States reports two or more diseases; this reaches 70.2% at age 80 years and older [4]. Analysis of Medicare claims data shows that two thirds of all beneficiaries aged older than 65 years have two or more chronic conditions, and one third have four or more [5]. Patients included in the Improving Mood—Promoting Access to Collaborative Treatment for late life depression (IMPACT) study, a randomized controlled trial on depression in the elderly, had an average of three to four physical diseases [6].

During the process of aging the general level of vulnerability increases, and age has become an indicator of health risks within the health care system. Although it seems reasonable to use biologic age as an indicator for health risks in the elderly, it is not a sensitive or specific indicator. The aging process different among people for genetic and environmental reasons; therefore, chronologic age becomes a poor indicator for biologic age. For that reason the value of chronologic age for medical prognosis and treatment decisions among the elderly is limited, and the concept of frailty becomes more important. In a sense, frailty is a proxy for the severity of the aging process in an individual, and is linked to, but distinct from, chronic diseases (comorbidity) and disability.

In the absence of a standard definition of frailty that is valid in different settings, any estimation of prevalence is tentative. The American Medical Association stated that as many as 40% of adults aged 80 years and older are frail [7]. In a sample of community-dwelling persons aged 65 years and older in the northern part of The Netherlands, the authors and colleagues [8] found a prevalence of frailty—measured by the Groningen Frailty Indicator (GFI)—of 32%. In the Longitudinal Aging Study Amsterdam (LASA), which included subjects ages 55 to 85 years, the prevalence of frailty—defined in a static and a dynamic way—ranged from 12% to 21% [9].

Frailty, comorbidity, and disability

Frailty is an aggregate expression of risks that result from age- or disease-associated physiologic accumulation of subthreshold decrements that affect multiple physiologic systems. Although the early stages of this process may be clinically silent, when the losses of reserve reach an aggregate threshold that leads to serious vulnerability, the syndrome may become detectable by looking at clinical, functional, behavioral, and biologic markers. Central to the clinical definition of frailty has been the concept that no single altered system defines this state, but that multiple systems must be involved. In this perspective, comorbidity is, by definition, related highly to frailty.

There also is a relationship between frailty, comorbidity, and disability. Disability is defined as difficulty or dependency in carrying out activities that are essential to independent living. It includes essential roles, such as tasks that are needed for self-care and living independently, and desired activities that are important to one's quality of life. Physical disability in late life primarily is an outcome of diseases and physiologic alterations with aging that is modified by social, economic, and behavioral factors as well as access to medical care. Although disability itself is an adverse health outcome, it also is a risk factor for other adverse events. Mobility disability predicts subsequent difficulty in instrumental activities of daily living (IADLs) and activities of daily living (ADLs) [10], and difficulty in these tasks is predictive of future dependency [11]. Additionally, disability—independent of its causes—is associated with an increased risk for mortality, hospitalization, the need for long-term care, and higher health care expenditures [12].

The epidemiologic relation between frailty, comorbidity, and disability has been documented well by Fried [13]. Using the standard definition of comorbidity in the Cardiovascular Health Study data, the presence of two or more diseases can identify a different, although overlapping, subset of the population than does the definition of frailty or the definition of disability (defined in this study as a difficulty in one or more ADLs). Overall, of the 368 participants (of 4317) who were frail, 27% reported disability in one ADL (with or without comorbidity), and 68% reported having two or more chronic conditions (with or without disability); 21% of those who were frail also were disabled and had comorbid disease (Fig. 1) [13].

Old or frail, what tells us more to guide treatment in the elderly?

Even the risk for individual mortality, which can be seen as the ultimate outcome of age and frailty [14], can be predicted better by frailty than by chronologic age [15]; however, a test of frailty versus chronologic age with self-management abilities (SMAs), a kind of coping skills, as an outcome measure was not available. To study the associations between frailty, SMAs, and age, the author and colleagues [16] first addressed the operationalizations of frailty and SMAs. The bundle of losses in resources that

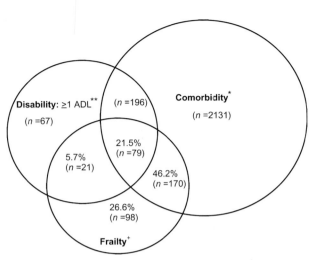

Fig. 1. Prevalences and overlaps of comorbidity, disability, and frailty among community-dwelling men and women 65 years and older participating in the Cardiovascular Health Study. (*From* Fried LP, Ferrucci L, Darer J, et al. Untangling the concepts of disability, frailty, and comorbidity: implications for improved targeting and care. J Gerontol A Biol Sci Med Sci 2004;59(3):255–63.)
Percents listed indicate the proportion among those who were frail (n = 368), who had comorbidity or disability, or neither. Total represented: 2762 participants who had comorbidity or disability or frailty. +n = 368 frail participants overall. *n = 2576 overall with two or more of the following nine diseases: myocardial infarction, angina, congestive heart failure, claudication, arthritis, cancer, diabetes, hypertension, chronic obstructive pulmonary disease. Of these, 249 (total) were also frail. **n = 363 overall with an activity of daily living disability; of these, 100 (total) were also frail.

constitutes frailty is expected to lead to the loss of SMAs. SMAs are abilities that are needed by an elderly person to prevent the loss of resources, to manage the decline and loss of resources, and to sustain well-being. These SMAs can be regarded as people's generative capacity to sustain well-being into old age. They play a key role in the complex adaptive systems that are needed for successful aging. Arguably, they are more important than is mortality as outcome measures of interventions, because they may be a more relevant concept for older people's well-being. Steverink and Lindenberg [17] addressed the topic of the key SMAs for older people, which are important for the management of their resources, such that their overall well-being is maintained or even improved, and losses are avoided or coped with adequately. Any intervention that is aimed at maintaining and improving well-being in elderly patients should incorporate aspects of SMAs. Based on a review of the literature on resources of well-being, six key SMAs could be specified. Moreover, with the help of a theory about human well-being—the social production function theory—explicit criteria for success (well-being and its dimensions) were specified. Both specifications led to the formulation of the theory of self-management of well-being, and both spec-ifications are considered to be essential for the design and evaluation of in-terventions. It is important to know which behavioral and cognitive SMAs are presumably essential for gaining and maintaining well-being (and are modifiable by interventions), and what well-being essentially refers to in terms of concrete dimensions that also can be addressed in interventions.

The GFI was developed as a short, simple questionnaire to be used as a case finder for elderly patients who would benefit from integrated (geriat-ric) care (Box 1). To be useful, the instrument should be able to predict poor outcome and it has to be related to complexity. The concept of complexity is elaborated further in the article by de Jonge and colleagues elsewhere in this issue. For clinical understanding, a differentiation is made between case complexity and care complexity. In clinical practice the negative pre-dictive value of such an indicator of complexity is the most important one. The author and colleagues investigated the predictive values of chronologic age and frailty in a large community sample of people aged 65 years and older that was drawn randomly from the register of six municipalities in the northern part of The Netherlands. People's generative capacity to sus-tain well-being—SMAs—was used as an outcome measure. The results show that when using chronologic age instead of frailty too many and too few people were selected. Moreover, frailty related more strongly ($\beta = -0.25$ to -0.39) to a decline in the SMAs than did chronologic age ($\beta = -0.06$ to -0.14). Chronologic age added little to the explained vari-ances of all outcomes after frailty had been included. The author and col-leagues also investigated the predictive power of the GFI in clinical studies. Patients older than the age of 65 years who had solid malignant tumors and underwent surgery as primary treatment of the disease (n = 83) at the University Medical Center Groningen were included in the study. The questionnaires used were the GFI, the European Organization for Re-search and Treatment of Cancer Quality of life Questionnaire (QLQ) C-30, the Charlson comorbidity index (CCMI), and the 10- to 30-day morbidity index. Linear regression showed that age, gender, and the CCMI could not predict QLQC-30 scales (physical function, role function, emotional func-tion) significantly 4 weeks and 3 months after surgery. When corrected for age, gender, and the CCMI, however, the GFI could predict most of the QLQC-30 scales significantly. The author and colleagues found clinical relevant and significant differences between the nonfrail and the frail groups after 4 weeks in mean scores on physical function (76 versus 48), role function (63 versus 32), emotional function (85 versus 66), social function (77 versus 63), and fatigue (37 versus 55). In the LASA study, a population-based cohort, frailty was defined in a similar way to the GFI. Frailty was an independent risk factor for a decline in physical func-tioning, institutionalization to a residential or nursing home, and mortality [18]. The investigators also demonstrated the importance of psychologic markers in the concept of frailty.

Box 1. The Groningen Frailty Indicator

Mobility
Is the patient able to carry out these tasks without any help?
(The use of help resources, such as walking stick, walking frame,
  wheelchair, is considered as independent)
  1. Shopping
  2. Walking around outside (around the house or to the
     neighbors)
  3. Dressing and undressing
  4. Going to the toilet
Physical fitness
  5. What mark does the patient give him/herself for physical
     fitness? (scale 0 to 10)
Vision
  6. Does the patient experience problems in daily life as
     a result of poor vision?
Hearing
  7. Does the patient experience problems in daily life because
     of difficulty hearing?
Nourishment
  8. During the last 6 months has the patient lost a lot of weight
     unwillingly? (3 kg in 1 month or 6 kg in 2 months)
Morbidity
  9. Does the patient take four or more different types of
     medicine?
Cognition (perception)
  10. Does the patient have any complaints about his/her
      memory or is the patient known to have a dementia
      syndrome?
Psychosocial
  11. Does the patient sometimes experience an emptiness
      around him/her?
  12. Does the patient sometimes miss people around him/her?
  13. Does the patient sometimes feel abandoned?
  14. Has the patient recently felt down-hearted or sad?
  15. Has the patient recently felt nervous or anxious?
Scoring:
  Questions 1–4: independent = 0; dependent = 1
  Question 5: 0–6 = 1; 7–10 = 0
  Questions 6–9: no = 0; yes = 1
  Question 10: no and sometimes = 0; yes = 1
  Questions 11–15: no = 0; sometimes and yes = 1

Relation between frailty and case complexity

In the article by de Jonge and colleagues elsewhere in this issue, arguments will be made to divide "complexity" into two clinical concepts—case- and care-complexity—with a linear relation. Generally speaking, the more complex the case, the more complex is the care that is needed. In complex medical situations there always will be a level of uncertainty that has to be managed in clinical care [19]. By disentangling complexity, opportunities are created to solve the most critical problems in view of the prognosis first. Elsewhere in this issue Stiefel and colleagues introduce a model for the assessment of case complexity: The INTERMED method (IM). The health risks/needs assessment with the IM allows the design of an integrated patient-oriented care plan. Because not every case, even in elderly patients, is complex and because assessments are costly—an interview and treatment planning take between 30 and 45 minutes—identifiers for case complexity are needed. This topic is discussed elsewhere in this issue (see the article by Huyse and colleagues). Arguments are made for the use of the GFI as an indicator for complex care needs in the elderly. The author examined the relation between the GFA and the IM in elderly inpatients. The study population consisted of 39 consecutive patients, at least 65 years of age, who were admitted to the Internal Medicine ward of the University Medical Center of Groningen. The age ranged from 65 to 92 years, with an average age of 79.6 years. Forty-one percent were men and 59% were women. The goal of the study was to demonstrate whether frailty is a suitable screening variable for complex elderly patients. Only one of the patients with a low GFI score (GFI = 3) had a high IM score (IM = 20). In other words, the screening recognized all complex patients. Out of the 25 patients with a high GFI score (> 3), 9 were complex and 16 were not. Out of the 16 patients with a GFI score of greater than 5, 9 were actually complex and 7 were not (Fig. 2).

In a clinical population of elderly patients, frailty, as measured by the GFI, seems to be a predictor for case complexity as measured by the INTERMED. In clinical practice the high negative predictive value of the frailty indicator is the most important one. Because frailty can exist on a subclinical level not every frail elderly patient will be complex nor will he have comorbidity or disabilities. Fries [20] demonstrated that there is an overlap between these concepts so that the frail elderly are at risk for being or becoming complex cases. Contrary to the general population there are few elderly patients in the hospital who have complex health risks but are not frail; however, taking into account that frailty usually precedes complexity, a high GFI tell us which patients are likely to need integrated care, immediately or in the future. Ideally, this group of patients would get care that is aimed at prevention, which would result in compression of disability and morbidity. Consequently, using frailty as an indicator to select older people who are at risk for unfavorable outcomes, and, as such—candidates for

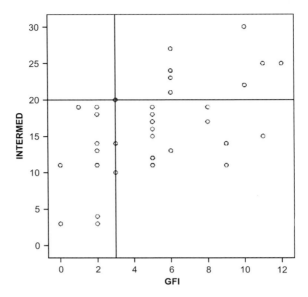

Fig. 2. Relation between INTERMED and GFI in elderly medical in-patients. $r = .55$.

integrated care—is, from a theoretic and empiric point of view, preferable to selecting people by their chronologic age. The GFI and the IM can help to redesign health care for elderly people with a primary focus on complexity, where relationships between parts are more important than the parts themselves, and minimum specifications for assessments, information flow, and multidisciplinary networks yield more creativity than do detailed plans [2] (see also the articles by de Jonge and colleagues, Huyse and colleagues, and Stiefel and colleagues elsewhere in this issue).

References

[1] Institute of Medicine. Crossing the quality chasm: a new health system for the 21st century. Committee on Quality of Health Care in America. National Academy Press: Washington DC; 2001.
[2] Plsek PE, Greenhalgh T. Complexity science. The challenge of complexity in health care. BMJ 2001;323(15):625–8.
[3] Verbrugge LM. Flies without wings. In: Carey R, Robin J-M, Michel J-P, et al, editors. Longevity and frailty. Heidelberg (Germany): Springer-Verlag; 2005. p. 67–81.
[4] Guralnik J, LaCroix A, Everett D, et al. Aging in the eighties: the prevalence of comorbidity and its association with disability. Advance Data From Vital and Health Statistics. Hyattsville (MD): National Center for Health Statistics; 1989.
[5] Anderson G. Testimony before the Subcommittee on Health of the House Committee on Ways and Means. Hearing on Promoting Disease Management in Medicare; 2002: Available at: http://waysandmeans.house.gov. Accessed June 2006.
[6] Unutzer J, Katon W, Callahan CM, et al. IMPACT. JAMA 2002;288(22):2835–45.
[7] American Medical Association white paper on elderly health. Report of the Council on Scientific Affairs. Arch Intern Med 1990;150(12):2459–72.

[8] Schuurmans H, Steverink N, Lindenberg S, et al. Old or frail: What tells us more? J Gerontol A Med Sci 2004;59:M962–5.
[9] Puts MTE, Lips P, Deeg DJH. Static and dynamic measures of frailty predicted decline in performance-based and self-reported physical functioning. J Clin Epidemiol 2005;58: 1188–98.
[10] Guralnik JM, Ferrucci L, Simonsick EM, et al. Lower-extremity function in persons over the age of 70 years as a predictor of subsequent disability. N Engl J Med 1995;332:556–61.
[11] Gill TM, Robison JT, Tinetti ME. Difficulty and dependence: two components of the disability continuum among community-living older persons. Ann Intern Med 1998;128:96–101.
[12] Fried LP, Kronmal RA, Newman AB, et al. Risk factors for 5-year mortality in older adults: the Cardiovascular Health Study. JAMA 1998;279:585–92.
[13] Fried LP, Ferrucci L, Darer J, et al. Untangling the concepts of disability, frailty, and comorbidity: implications for improved targeting and care. J Gerontol A Biol Sci Med Sci 2004; 59(3):255–63.
[14] Morley GE, Perry HM, Miller DK. Editorial: something about frailty. J Gerontol A Biol Sci Med Sci 2002;57(11):M698–704.
[15] Mitnitski AB, Mogilner AJ, MacKnight C, et al. The mortality rate as a function of accumulated deficits in a frailty index. Mech Ageing Dev 2002;123:1457–60.
[16] Steverink N, Lindenberg S, Slaets JPJ. How to understand and improve older people's self-management of wellbeing. Eur J Ageing 2005;2:235–44.
[17] Steverink N, Lindenberg S. Which social needs are important for subjective well-being? What happens to them with aging? Psychol Aging 2006;21(2):281–90.
[18] Puts MTE, Lips P, Ribbe MW, et al. The effect of frailty on residential/nursing home admissions in The Netherlands independent of chronic diseases and functional limitations. European Journal of Ageing 2005;2(4):264–74.
[19] Wilson T, Holt T. Complexity science. Complexity and clinical care. BMJ 2001;323(22): 685–8.
[20] Fries JF. Aging, natural death, and the compression of morbidity. N Engl J Med 1980; 303(3):130–5.

ELSEVIER
SAUNDERS

Med Clin N Am 90 (2006) 603–626

THE MEDICAL
CLINICS
OF NORTH AMERICA

Symptoms, Syndromes, and the Value of Psychiatric Diagnostics in Patients Who Have Functional Somatic Disorders

Kurt Kroenke, MD[a,b,*],
Judith G.M. Rosmalen, PhD, MA[c,d]

[a]Department of Medicine, Indiana University School of Medicine
[b]Regenstrief Institute, RG-6, 1050 Wishard Boulevard, Indianapolis, IN 46202, USA
[c]Department of Psychiatry, University Medical Center Groningen, University of Groningen,
Hanzeplein 1, 9713 GZ Groningen, The Netherlands
[d]Graduate School for Experimental Psychopathology, The Netherlands

The epidemiology of physical symptoms has been reviewed recently [1,2]. Symptoms account for more than half of all outpatient encounters or, in the United States alone, nearly 400 million clinic visits annually. About one half of these are pain complaints (eg, headache, chest pain, abdominal pain, joint pains), one quarter are upper respiratory (eg, cough, sore throat, ear or nasal symptoms), and the remainder are neither pain nor upper respiratory symptoms (eg, fatigue, dizziness, palpitations). About three fourths of outpatients who present with physical complaints experience improvement within 2 weeks, whereas 20% to 25% are chronic or recurrent [3,4]. Symptoms that are self-limiting (viral respiratory illnesses) or explained readily (eg, angina pectoris in the patient who has classic symptoms and known cardiovascular risk factors, or asthma in the patient who has acute dyspnea and wheezing) are not particularly perplexing. Rather, it is the symptoms that are unexplained and often chronic that are frustrating for providers and patients and costly for the health care system.

This article highlights (1) an overview of unexplained symptoms and somatization; (2) limitations of the *Diagnostic and Statistical Manual of Mental Disorders, Fourth Edition* (DSM-IV) in classifying somatoform disorders; (3) predictors of psychiatric comorbidity in patients with physical symptoms; and (4) measuring and managing symptoms.

* Corresponding author. Regenstrief Institute, RG-6, 1050 Wishard Boulevard, Indianapolis, IN 46202.
E-mail address: kkroenke@regenstrief.org (K. Kroenke).

0025-7125/06/$ - see front matter
doi:10.1016/j.mcna.2006.04.003

Unexplained symptoms and somatization

Studies in the general population as well as primary care and specialty clinic patients have shown that at least one third to one half of symptoms are medically unexplained [2]. One reason for this absence of medical explanation is the frequent lack of objective findings on physical examination or diagnostic testing. Another reason may be the misleading nature of objective findings in certain patients (eg, the cardiac flow murmur that has no causal connection to the patient's atypical chest pain or shortness of breath). Several symptom categories are more descriptive than etiologic. Mechanical low back pain, nonulcer dyspepsia, myofascial pain syndromes, and costochondritis are only a few examples of diagnoses with which symptomatic patients are labeled commonly, but for which diagnostic criteria typically are vague. In one of the few instances where this has been studied rigorously, it was found that three experts who reviewed the same data on the same patients and used explicit diagnostic criteria demonstrated only modest interobserver agreement on classifying the cause of dizziness in specific patients [5]. Likewise, the distinction between migraine and tension headache is not always clear-cut, which leads some experts to argue for a continuum theory of migraine on one end of the spectrum and tension headache on the other, rather than a dichotomous classification [6]. This diagnostic heterogeneity among clinicians who evaluate the same symptoms leads to considerable variability in diagnostic testing and treatment approaches [7].

Proliferation of diagnostic testing has yielded a burgeoning number of false positive results that may be linked mistakenly to nonspecific symptoms. One example is the attribution of low back pain to disc abnormalities that are seen on MRI, a diagnosis that is complicated by the fact that 40% of asymptomatic controls had some degree of disc abnormality on MRI [8]. In fact, radiographic abnormalities in an important fraction of the general population has led to a new term, "incidentaloma" [9,10]. Other examples include the overdiagnosis of Lyme disease in a patient who has fatigue, musculoskeletal pain, and low-level antibody titers [11,12] or "subclinical hypothyroidism" in a patient who has vague symptoms and borderline elevations of thyroid-stimulating hormone. Meador [13] warned of the overinterpretation of laboratory (as well as physical) findings in his classic essay, "The Art and Science of Nondisease."

Experts do not agree entirely on how to define somatization. There are two competing definitions. The first maintains simply that somatization is the process whereby individuals experience and report physical symptoms that, after appropriate investigation, cannot be explained fully by a known general medical condition. The second definition requires the absence of an explanatory medical condition and the presence of psychologic factors that are causing or contributing to the symptom. Confirming that psychologic factors are the actual cause of physical symptoms, rather than merely a consequence or coexisting condition, may not be easy. Also, somatizing patients may resist efforts to attribute their symptoms to nonphysical causes strenu-ously, which makes it difficult for the practitioner to explore emotional un-derpinnings openly or offer psychologic treatments.

Although a chronic history of unexplained symptoms builds the strongest case for somatization, follow-up studies of selected symptoms, such as fa-tigue, dizziness, chest pain, abdominal pain, palpitations, and back pain, have confirmed the clinician's initial judgment that a symptom is unex-plained usually is correct and that the delayed emergence of serious diagno-ses that were not suspected initially is rare [14–20].

Somatization is associated with increased health care use, functional im-pairment, provider dissatisfaction, and psychiatric comorbidity. Somatizing patients disproportionately use health care resources, and experience high rates of clinic and emergency room visits, excessive diagnostic testing, fre-quent subspecialty referrals, and polypharmacy because of multiple thera-peutic trials. Moreover, care of the somatizing patient frequently is disjointed because of the number and diversity of health care providers that are involved. This fragmentation of care makes it especially difficult to control medication prescribing, test ordering, and other medical costs.

Medically unexplained symptoms are a major public health problem. The lack of objective findings leads to diagnostic heterogeneity among clinicians who evaluate the same somatic symptom. In case of a chronic history of un-explained symptoms, the presence of a somatoform disorder might be sus-pected, in which psychologic factors are causing or contributing to the symptoms.

Diagnosis of somatoform disorders: limitations of the *Diagnostic and Statistical Manual of Mental Disorders* diagnostic system

The first edition of the DSM was published in 1952. Although the first two editions of the DSM were based mainly on psychodynamic etiologic principles, since the *Diagnostic and Statistical Manual of Mental Disorders, Third Edition* (DSM-III), which was published in the early 1980s, the edi-tions have been based increasingly on clusters of symptoms that were de-rived primarily from clinical observation and epidemiologic research. Despite this development, criteria for DSM diagnoses are not established on a truly empiric basis; instead, expert consensus is used. Expert consensus remains an opinion rather than the objective truth. Consequently, the DSM diagnostic system has been criticized extensively.

Somatoform disorders form no exception to this rule. The category of so-matoform disorders first was included in DSM-III as a group of diagnoses that was characterized by the presentation of physical symptoms that sug-gest a medical condition. In DSM-IV, the somatoform category is composed of the subcategories of somatization disorder (SD), undifferentiated somato-form disorder, hypochondriasis, body dysmorphic disorder, conversion dis-order, and pain disorder (diagnostic criteria are summarized in Table 1). As

Table 1
Diagnostic and Statistical Manual of Mental Disorders, Fourth Edition diagnostic criteria for somatoform disorders

Disorders	Diagnostic Criteria
Somatization disorder	A. A history of many physical complaints beginning before age 30 years that occur over a period of several years and result in treatment being sought or significant impairment in social, occupational, or other important areas of functioning.
	B. Each of the following criteria must have been met, with individual symptoms occurring at any time during the course of the disturbance:
	(1) Four pain symptoms: a history of pain related to at least four different sites or functions (eg, head, abdomen, back, joints, extremities, chest, rectum, during menstruation, during sexual intercourse, or during urination)
	(2) Two gastrointestinal symptoms: a history of at least two gastrointestinal symptoms other than pain (eg, nausea, bloating, vomiting other than during pregnancy, diarrhea, or intolerance of several different foods)
	(3) One sexual symptom: a history of at least one sexual or reproductive symptom other than pain (eg, sexual indifference, erectile or ejaculatory dysfunction, irregular menses, excessive menstrual bleeding, vomiting throughout pregnancy)
	(4) One pseudoneurologic symptom: a history of at least one symptom or deficit suggesting a neurologic condition not limited to pain (conversion symptoms, such as impaired coordination or balance, paralysis, or localized weakness; difficulty swallowing or lump in throat; aphonia; urinary retention; hallucinations; loss of touch or pain sensation; double vision; blindness; deafness; seizures; dissociative symptoms, such as amnesia; or loss of consciousness other than fainting)
	C. Either (1) or (2):
	(1) After appropriate investigation, each of the symptoms in criterion B cannot be explained fully by a known general medical condition or the direct effects of a substance (eg, a drug of abuse, a medication)
	(2) When there is a related general medical condition, the physical complaints or resulting social or occupational impairment are in excess of what would be expected from the history, physical examination, or laboratory findings
	D. The symptoms are not feigned or produced intentionally (as in factitious disorder or malingering).

Undifferentiated somatoform disorder

A. One or more physical complaints (eg, fatigue, loss of appetite, gastrointestinal or urinary complaints)

B. Either (1) or (2):

(1) After appropriate investigation, the symptoms cannot be explained fully by a known general medical condition or the direct effects of a substance (eg, a drug of abuse, a medication)

(2) When there is a related general medical condition, the physical complaints or resulting social or occupational impairment is in excess of what would be expected from the history, physical examination, or laboratory findings

C. The symptoms cause clinically significant distress or impairment in social, occupational, or other important areas of functioning

D. The duration of the disturbance is at least 6 months

E. The disturbance is not better accounted for by another mental disorder (eg, another somatoform disorder, sexual dysfunction, mood disorder, anxiety disorder, sleep disorder, or psychotic disorder)

F. The symptom is not produced or feigned intentionally (as in factitious disorder or malingering)

Hypochondriasis

A. Preoccupation with fears of having, or the idea that one has, a serious disease based on the person's misinterpretation of bodily symptoms

B. The preoccupation persists despite appropriate medical evaluation and reassurance

C. The belief in criterion A is not of delusional intensity (as in delusional disorder, somatic type) and is not restricted to a circumscribed concern about appearance (as in body dysmorphic disorder)

D. The preoccupation causes clinically significant distress or impairment in social, occupational, or other important areas of functioning

E. The duration of the disturbance is at least 6 months

F. The preoccupation is not accounted for better by generalized anxiety disorder, obsessive-compulsive disorder, panic disorder, a major depressive episode, separation anxiety, or another somatoform disorder

Body dysmorphic disorder

A. Preoccupation with an imagined defect in appearance. If a slight physical anomaly is present, the person's concern is markedly excessive.

B. The preoccupation causes clinically significant distress or impairment in social, occupational, or other important areas of functioning

C. The preoccupation is not accounted for better by another mental disorder (eg, dissatisfaction with body shape and size in anorexia nervosa)

(continued on next page)

Table 1 (*continued*)

Disorders	Diagnostic Criteria
Conversion disorder	A. One or more symptoms or deficits affecting voluntary motor or sensory function that suggest a neurologic or other general medical condition B. Psychologic factors are judged to be associated with the symptom or deficit because the initiation or exacerbation of the symptom or deficit is preceded by conflicts or other stressors C. The symptom or deficit is not produced or feigned intentionally (as in factitious disorder or malingering) D. The symptom or deficit cannot, after appropriate investigation, be explained fully by a general medical condition, or by the direct effects of a substance, or as a culturally sanctioned behavior or experience E. The symptom or deficit causes clinically significant distress or impairment in social, occupational, or other important areas of functioning or warrants medical evaluation F. The symptom or deficit is not limited to pain or sexual dysfunction, does not occur exclusively during the course of somatization disorder, and is not better accounted for by another mental disorder
Pain disorder	A. Pain in one or more anatomic sites is the predominant focus of the clinical presentation and is of sufficient severity to warrant clinical attention B. The pain causes clinically significant distress or impairment in social, occupational, or other important areas of functioning C. Psychologic factors are judged to have an important role in the onset, severity, exacerbation, or maintenance of the pain D. The symptom or deficit is not produced or feigned intentionally (as in factitious disorder or malingering) E. The pain is not accounted for better by a mood, anxiety, or psychotic disorder and does not meet criteria for dyspareunia

Adapted from the American Psychiatric Association. Diagnostic and Statistical Manual of Mental Disorders DSM-IV, 2004; with permission.

is the case for other DSM diagnostic categories, the overall concept of soma-toform disorders and its subcategories have remained a focus of criticism de-spite subsequent modifications [21,22]. The main problem of DSM seems to be the implicit assumption that mental disorders are disease entities that can be defined by operationalized sets of symptom criteria; however, this as-sumption is questionable and comes with potentially harmful side effects. Three of these side effects are discussed: problems identifying the border between disorder and normality, proliferation of new diagnoses, and magni-fication of comorbidity, thereby focusing on the diagnosis of somatoform disorders.

Border problems between disorder and normality

It is unclear how to distinguish between mental disorder and nondisor-der problems of living. The main assumption of a categorical diagnostic model—that diagnoses have an identifiable separation from normality—implies that the distribution of clinical features of the phenotypes of diseases states must have discontinuities; however, many of the DSM diag-noses most likely represent entities in which cut-off points have been superimposed arbitrarily on variables that seem to be distributed continu-ously in the population. For example, a variety of studies has found that personality disorders merge with normality [23]. Despite the fact that re-searchers have been unable to identify a qualitative distinction between normal functioning and mental disorder, DSM-IV provides specific and ex-plicit rules for the number and severity of sign and symptom criteria that are required for diagnosing a "case" of mental disorder. The thresholds for diagnosis that are provided in DSM-IV remain largely unexplained and weakly justified [24].

Somatoform disorders are no exception to this shortcoming of DSM. Es-cobar and colleagues [25] reviewed the criteria for the diagnosis of SD in the subsequent DSM editions: from 25 unexplained somatic symptoms from a list of 59 in addition to attitudinal features in DSM-I; to a symptom count of 14 (men, DSM-III) or 16 (women, DSM-III) followed by 13 (both gen-ders, DSM-IIIR) from a list of 37 symptoms; to the current criteria of 8 symptoms coming from four designated organ systems in DSM-IV. The modifications already indicate the arbitrary distinction between a case and a noncase. As observed for other psychiatric phenotypes, the number of so-matic symptoms that a person reports is distributed continuously in the gen-eral population, and the diagnosis merely represents an extreme on a continuum of distress [26]. There seems to be no qualitative difference be-tween patients who meet the criteria for the diagnosis of SD, and those who only have some symptoms but do not meet the formal criteria. Even the di-agnostic criteria of disorders that are not based on symptom counts, are, by definition, arbitrary. Consider, for example, hypochondriasis: no norms exist for levels of illness worry that are appropriate for a patient's medical condition [27].

The arbitrary criteria for distinguishing between the presence and absence of a mental disorder obviously result in two main diagnostic problems: false positives and false negatives. Because symptoms of many mental disorders commonly occur in persons who do not have a psychiatric disorder as normal reactions to psychosocial stress, avoiding false positives is difficult. The solution for this problem is the inclusion of the clinical significance criterion (eg, "the disturbance causes clinically significant distress or impairment in social, occupational, or other important areas of functioning") to a large number of disorders in DSM-IV. The clinical significance criterion attempts to minimize false positive diagnoses in situations in which the symptom criteria do not necessarily indicate pathology. This criterion has been criticized on several grounds [28]. The main criticism is that many of the diagnostic symptom criteria are associated inherently with significant impairment, so that the clinical significance criterion is redundant, and therefore, does not affect the definition of a case. In case of somatoform disorders, a study in a primary care setting demonstrated that when the new DSM-IV criterion of moderate to severe clinical impairment was ignored, the prevalence of somatoform disorders increased from 16% to 22% [29]. This indicated that the clinical significance criterion might avoid false positive diagnoses of somatoform disorders.

The clinical significance criterion increases the chance of false negative diagnoses (ie, failure to diagnose psychiatric disorders that are present), or subthreshold conditions. There is much evidence to support the notion that subthreshold conditions are important public health problems; however, given the problems with clarifying diagnostic boundaries between normality and (suprathreshold) DSM disorders, it is logical that it is even more difficult to define subthreshold diagnoses. Abridged SD and multisomatoform disorder have been proposed as less restrictive somatoform disorders, and both were demonstrated to be associated with excess functional impairment and health care use [26,30].

Proliferation of new diagnoses

One of the most striking features of every new edition of the DSM is the addition of a large number of new psychiatric disorders. Fig. 1 shows the numbers of diagnoses included in the DSM editions: 106 in DSM-I (1952), 182 in DSM-II (1968), 265 in DSM-III (1980), 292 in DSM-IIIR (1987), and 365 in DSM-IV (1994). There is a close relationship between the year of publication of a DSM edition and number of diagnoses that is included in that edition (in which year of publication explains as much as 98% of the variance in number of diagnoses). By extrapolating this relationship to DSM-V, which is expected to be published in 2012, it can be estimated that this edition will include 457 diagnoses.

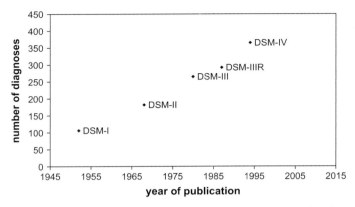

Fig. 1. Number of diagnoses of psychiatric disorders in DSM editions as a function of year of publication.

It is questionable whether the new diagnostic entities that are added to every new edition reflect an enhanced understanding of the etiology of psychiatric disorders. In case of somatoform disorders, most of the subcategories remain controversial. Several of the somatoform subcategories also could be regarded as specific manifestations of psychiatric diagnoses from other diagnostic categories. For example, based on the phenomenological similarities with several anxiety disorders [31], it could be argued that hypochondriasis should be regarded as an anxiety disorder that happens to focus on health issues [22]. In the same line, body dysmorphic disorder merely might be a form of obsessive-compulsive disorder in which the compulsive ideas and behaviors (mirror checking) and obsessive thoughts concern the body [32]. Conversion disorder could be reunited with dissociative disorder, because similar psychologic processes seem to underlie these disorders, despite their descriptive differences [28]. SD might be better regarded as a combination of personality disorder and anxiety and depressive syndromes [33]. Significant difficulties were found in differentiating between the diagnoses of undifferentiated somatoform disorder and pain disorder in a sample of 127 patients [34]. Independent of the major presenting complaint, most of the patients had multiple pain and nonpain symptoms. The investigators concluded that the differential diagnosis relies on whether the investigator judges the number of symptoms or the preoccupation with pain as the most important factor for diagnosis [34]. In conclusion, it is unclear whether the existing somatoform disorders truly are independent diagnostic entities.

Additionally, despite this proliferation of presumed psychiatric diagnostic entities, DSM diagnoses still do not cover common clinical cases adequately. To solve this problem, DSM includes "not otherwise specific" (NOS) categories, into which atypical conditions or conditions that do not meet the full criteria for a specific mental disorder are placed. Undifferentiated somatoform disorder was placed alongside somatoform disorder–NOS in DSM-IIIR to diagnose patients who had a somatoform disorder that did not fit into one of the specific DSM-III categories [22]. Subsequent studies demonstrated that undifferentiated somatoform disorder was the most common somatoform disorder [29], which illustrates the limitations of the existing DSM diagnostic categories.

Magnification of comorbidity

Given the proliferation of psychiatric diagnoses, it is not surprising that psychiatric comorbidity also is encountered frequently. High rates of psychiatric comorbidity have been observed in numerous clinical and epidemiologic samples [35–39].

As can be anticipated, somatoform disorders also are accompanied frequently by other mental disorders. A high comorbidity of somatoform disorders and especially anxiety or depressive disorders was a common finding in previous studies [25,40]. A recent study in a primary care setting demonstrated that 26% of patients who had a somatoform disorder also had an anxiety or depressive disorder. Conversely, 54% of all patients who had an anxiety or depressive disorder also had a somatoform disorder [29]. Several investigators have studied psychiatric comorbidity for the specific subcategories of somatoform disorders in the community, primary care patients, and psychiatric patients. Concerning SD, depressive disorders have been diagnosed in 55% to 94% of patients who have SD, panic disorder has been diagnosed in 26% to 45% of patients who have SD, and phobic disorder has been diagnosed in 25% to 39% of patients who have SD [41]; the higher rates usually are found in psychiatric patients. Of patients who had SD in the primary care setting, 34% met the diagnostic criteria for generalized anxiety disorder [41]. Additionally, excessive co-occurrence of personality disorders has been found; structured interviews documented that 23% of patients who had SD in the primary care setting had one personality disorder and 37% had two or more personality disorders [42]. The four most frequently identified personality disorders were avoidance (27%), paranoia (21%), self-defeating (19%), and obsessive-compulsive (17%) [42]. Studies in primary care outpatients who had hypochondriasis demonstrated that 62% to 88% had one or more additional clinical psychiatric disorder; the overlap was greatest with depressive (44%–55% for any depressive disorder) and anxiety (22%–86% for any anxiety disorder) disorders [31]. Likewise, patients who have body dysmorphic disorder have a current prevalence of 59% for major depression and a lifetime prevalence of 83%; they also have a 35% lifetime prevalence for primary social phobia and an 11% lifetime prevalence for panic disorder [32].

This degree of overlap exists despite the fact that several DSM diagnoses include hierarchical criteria to ensure that diagnoses are mutually exclusive. Consider, for example, the DSM-IV definition of generalized anxiety disorder. The essential feature of this disorder is excessive anxiety and worry that occurs for a certain period of time about several events or activities. The diagnostic criteria pose restrictions to the focus of the anxiety and worry; it should not be confined to features of another clinical psychiatric disorder, such as having a panic attack (eg, in panic disorder), being embarrassed in public (eg, social phobia), being contaminated (eg, obsessive-compulsive disorder), being away from home or close relatives (eg, separation anxiety disorder), gaining weight (eg, anorexia nervosa), having multiple physical complaints (eg, SD), or having a serious illness (eg, hypochondriasis), and the anxiety and worry should not occur exclusively during post-traumatic stress disorder. Without these exclusion criteria, the overlap between somatoform disorders and other DSM disorders would be even more extensive.

In the case of somatoform disorders, there is a special problem concerning the exclusion criteria; it is unclear whether functional somatic syndromes, such as chronic fatigue syndrome or fibromyalgia, count as exclusions. This may result in artificial comorbidity because patients may be classified as having a nonpsychiatric medical disorder (eg, irritable bowel syndrome) and a somatoform disorder (eg, undifferentiated somatoform disorder or pain disorder) for the same somatic symptoms [22]. Several investigators concluded that a substantial overlap exists between the individual functional somatic syndromes, and that the similarities between them (in case definition, reported symptoms, and in nonsymptom association [eg, patients' sex, outlook, and response to treatment]) outweigh the differences [43–45]. It seems that the difference between somatoform disorders and functional somatic syndromes depends mainly on the investigator (functional somatic syndromes are used widely in primary care and general medicine, whereas somatoform disorders are used in psychiatric settings).

A second diagnostic problem is the criterion excluding symptoms that are "better accounted for by a general medical condition." Evidence from multiple studies indicate that even symptoms that might be attributable to a comorbid physical disorder may not be explained fully by that disorder. Examples include

Exercise tolerance in some patients who have chronic obstructive pulmonary disease may correlate better with depression than with abnormalities on spirometric testing [46].

Diabetic symptoms may correlate more strongly with psychologic factors than with the degree of glucose control [47,48].

Palpitations correlate with stress and tendencies to amplify somatic symptoms, rather than cardiac ectopy, on electrocardiographic monitoring [49].

Angina burden in patients who have heart disease is predicted more by depression severity than by findings on echocardiographic stress testing [50].

Cognitive complaints following coronary artery bypass surgery correlate
better with measures of depression and anxiety than with neuropsychologic test results [51].
Among patients who have cancer or are HIV positive, unexplained symptoms are common and are associated strongly with depression [52,53].

This "nonspecificity" of apparently disease-specific symptoms was highlighted in a recent study of nearly 3500 patients who were 60 years and older
and attended a primary care clinic [54]. As shown in Fig. 2, chest pain was
only moderately more prevalent in patients who had heart disease compared
with other diseases; this finding also was noted for other conditions (eg, joint
pain and arthritis, dyspnea and pulmonary disease).

In summary, the diagnosis of DSM somatoform disorders in patients
who have medically unexplained symptoms is complicated. Problems include identifying the border between disorder and normality. Moreover, diagnostic proliferation and high rates of comorbidity among patients who
have DSM-diagnosed mental disorders suggest that symptoms that are associated with psychopathology do not divide easily into mutually exclusive
categories. The nonspecificity of current therapies illustrates this; although
the number of diagnoses continues to increase, the main classes of drugs
are used increasingly across diagnostic categories. For example, selective serotonin reuptake inhibitor medications, although initially regarded as antidepressants, were reported to be part of the treatment of many anxiety
disorders, schizophrenia (negative symptoms), and anorexia nervosa
[55,56]. The use of atypical antipsychotics is well established in bipolar disorder, schizophrenia, and psychosis in general, but it also has been successful in the treatment of psychotic and behavioral disorders in dementia of
various   types,   refractory   obsessive-compulsive   disorder,   pervasive

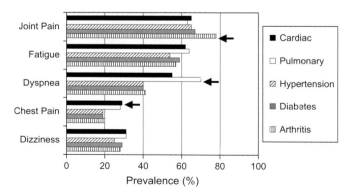

Fig. 2. "Nonspecificity" of apparently disease-specific symptoms, as highlighted in a prevalence
study of physical symptoms in 3498 patients who were 60 years and older and attended a primary care clinic. The prevalence of each symptom is shown in patients who have one of five
medical conditions: cardiac disease, pulmonary disease, hypertension, diabetes, and arthritis.
Arrows denote the disease for which a particular symptom is expected to be more prevalent.

developmental disorder, stuttering and Tourette's syndrome, refractory depression, and borderline personality disorder [57]. The options for psychotherapy are restricted to cognitive-behavioral therapy (and its derivates) and psychodynamic therapy. Thus, new diagnostic categories may not lead to the development of more specific therapies. It is obvious that a multidisciplinary approach is necessary in patients who have somatoform disorders. The first prerequisite is to identify the somatizing patient, and thus, to recognize the predictors of psychiatric comorbidity in patients who have physical complaints.

Predictors of psychiatric comorbidity

Depressive, anxiety, and somatoform disorders are the three most common comorbid psychiatric conditions in patients who present with physical complaints [2,58–63]. At least one third to one half of all physical complaints are unexplained medically; a depressive disorder can be diagnosed 50% to 60% of the time and an anxiety disorder can be diagnosed 40% to 50% of the time, regardless of the symptom. Also, physical symptoms are unexplained medically in at least one third of patients who are referred to specialty clinics [64]. Among patients who were referred to three specialty clinics (gastroenterology, rheumatology, neurology), depression was present in one quarter to one third of patients in each clinic, and depressed patients were only about one-fourth as likely to have a physical diagnosis established as an explanation for the symptoms that triggered their referral.

Although the specific type of symptom is not particularly important in terms of predicting depression or anxiety, the number of symptoms is. As shown in Fig. 3, there is a strong relationship between the number of physical symptoms that is endorsed by patients as currently bothersome and the likelihood of a coexisting depressive or anxiety disorder [59,60]. Thus, the number of symptoms might be an appropriate identifier ("red flag") for patients who require an integrated analysis of their complaints (see the article by Huyse and colleagues elsewhere in this issue). This relationship is for total symptom count—medically explained and unexplained. Although limiting the count to unexplained symptoms strengthens the relationship with depression and anxiety [26,59,62], the total symptom count itself is a powerful predictor and does not require the clinician to go through the time-consuming and subjective process of adjudicating the somatoform nature of each individual symptom. Besides the simple total number of symptoms, other symptom count thresholds that predict psychiatric comorbidity are three or more unexplained bothersome symptoms with at least a several year history of somatization [30], pain in at least two different regions of the body, and multiple functional somatic syndromes [65].

One common question is "What is the cause of somatic symptoms in the person who has multiple medical conditions?". Couldn't the person who has

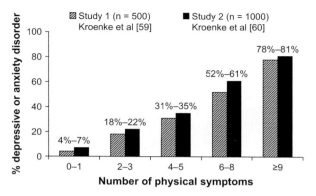

Fig. 3. Increased likelihood of depressive or anxiety disorder as the number of physical symptoms endorsed on a 15-symptom checklist increased in two primary care studies that involved 500 and 1000 patients.

heart disease, chronic lung disease, esophageal reflux, and osteoarthritis be bothered by multiple physical symptoms? Although this is true theoretically, the reality is that patients who have multiple medical problems typically endorse only a limited number of symptoms as currently bothersome on a symptom checklist; when offered a menu, they focus on a few predominant complaints. Physical symptom count has a much stronger relationship with depressive and anxiety disorders than with the number of medical disorders. A second question is "What is the possibility of a single polysymptomatic disease in someone who reports multiple symptoms?". The fact is that depression and anxiety are exceptionally common, whereas these multisystem diseases are infrequent in primary care and usually have other objective manifestations besides symptoms.

Besides unexplained or multiple symptoms, Box 1 summarizes some of the factors that increase the likelihood of a concurrent psychiatric disorder in the individual who has physical symptoms. Chronicity or recurrence of symptoms is one such factor. Also, the clinician's own reaction to the visit is another predictor [66–68]. One out of six primary care visits is perceived as "difficult" by the physician; patients who trigger such difficult encounters are three times more likely to have a depressive or anxiety disorder and are nine times more likely to have a somatoform disorder. Four predictors that constitute the "S4 model" (recent stress, high symptom count, high symptom severity, and low self-rated health) are assessed easily. The likelihood of a depressive or anxiety disorder with 0, 1, 2, 3, or 4 of these S4 predictors is 8%, 16%, 43%, 69%, and 94%, respectively [2,60]. Finally, other predictors of psychiatric comorbidity in patients with physical complaints include high health care use [69] and medication history, including polypharmacy; failure to respond to numerous medication trials for the same symptom; and intolerance of multiple medications, which Barsky and colleagues [70] referred to as the "nocebo" effect.

Box 1. Predictors of psychiatric comorbidity (especially depressive, anxiety, or somatoform disorders) in patients who have physical symptoms

Unexplained symptom after the clinician's initial assessment
Multiple symptoms
    Three or more unexplained symptoms
    Pain symptoms in two or more regions of the body
    Multiple functional somatic syndromes
Chronic or recurrent symptoms
Frequent health care use (clinic or emergency department visits; hospitalizations)
Medication history
    Polypharmacy (especially for symptoms)
    Failure to respond to multiple medication trials for the same symptom
    Intolerance of multiple medications ("nocebo" effect)
    Difficult encounter (as perceived by clinician)
Number of S4 predictors
    Stress in past week
    Symptom count high (>5 on the Patient Health Questionnaire 15-symptom checklist)
    Self-rated health is low (fair to poor)
    Severity of symptom is high (>5 on a 10-point scale where 0 is none and 10 is unbearable)

Measuring symptoms

It is clear that measuring physical and depressive and anxiety symptoms is useful in sorting out the number and types of somatic symptoms and the co-occurrence of psychiatric comorbidity. There are several case-finding measures for depression, none of which is clearly superior [71]. There are fewer practical measures for anxiety or somatoform disorders. The Patient Health Questionnaire (PHQ), which has five scales for assessing depressive, anxiety, somatoform, alcohol, and eating disorders, is a multidisorder diagnostic measure that was designed for the efficient evaluation of medical patients [72,73]. Fig. 4 shows the first page of the PHQ, which consists of the somatic and depressive symptom scales. The nine-item depression scale is known as the PHQ-9, and the 13-item somatic symptom scale combined with the fatigue and sleep items from the depression scale constitute the PHQ-15.

Detailed information regarded validation and scoring has been reported [74–76]. Briefly, the PHQ-9 has four response options for each depressive symptom, which can be scored as 0, 1, 2, and 3; the total PHQ-9 score

1. **During the <u>last 4 weeks</u>, how much have you been bothered by any of the following problems?**

	Not bothered	Bothered a little	Bothered a lot
a. Stomach pain..	☐	☐	☐
b. Back pain...	☐	☐	☐
c. Pain in your arms, legs, or joints (knees, hips, etc.)...	☐	☐	☐
d. Menstrual cramps or other problems with your periods..	☐	☐	☐
e. Pain or problems during sexual intercourse.............	☐	☐	☐
f. Headaches..	☐	☐	☐
g. Chest pain..	☐	☐	☐
h. Dizziness..	☐	☐	☐
i. Fainting spells...	☐	☐	☐
j. Feeling your heart pound or race............................	☐	☐	☐
k. Shortness of breath...	☐	☐	☐
l. Constipation, loose bowels, or diarrhea..................	☐	☐	☐
m. Nausea, gas, or indigestion..................................	☐	☐	☐

2. **Over the <u>last 2 weeks</u>, how often have you been bothered by any of the following problems?**

	Not at all	Several days	More than half the days	Nearly every day
a. Little interest or pleasure in doing things......................	☐	☐	☐	☐
b. Feeling down, depressed, or hopeless........................	☐	☐	☐	☐
c. Trouble falling or staying asleep, or sleeping too much..	☐	☐	☐	☐
d. Feeling tired or having little energy............................	☐	☐	☐	☐
e. Poor appetite or overeating..	☐	☐	☐	☐
f. Feeling bad about yourself — or that you are a failure or have let yourself or your family down........................	☐	☐	☐	☐
g. Trouble concentrating on things, such as reading the newspaper or watching television............................	☐	☐	☐	☐
h. Moving or speaking so slowly that other people could have noticed? Or the opposite — being so fidgety or restless that you have been moving around a lot more than usual..	☐	☐	☐	☐
i. Thoughts that you would be better off dead or of hurting yourself in some way...	☐	☐	☐	☐

If you checked off <u>any</u> problems on this questionnaire, how <u>difficult</u> have these problems made it for you to do your work, take care of things at home, or get along with other people?

Not difficult at all	Somewhat difficult	Very difficult	Extremely difficult
☐	☐	☐	☐

Developed by Drs. Robert L. Spitzer, Janet B.W. Williams, Kurt Kroenke and colleagues, with an educational grant from Pfizer Inc. For research information, contact Dr. Kroenke at kkroenke@regenstrief.org

The names PRIME-MD® and PRIME-MD TODAY® are trademarks of Pfizer, Inc.

Fig. 4. Somatic symptom and depression modules of the Patient Health Questionnaire. (Reproduced with permission from Pfizer, Inc.)

ranges from 0 to 27. Cutpoints of 5, 10, 15, and 20 represent mild, moderate, moderately severe, and severe depression, respectively. A decline of 5 points or more represents a clinically significant improvement, and a score of less than 5 represents remission. The 13 somatic symptoms have three response options that can be scored 0, 1, and 2. When included in the PHQ-15 score, the fatigue and sleep items from the PHQ-9 depression scale are also scored as 0 ("not at all"), 1 ("several days"), and 2 ("more than half the days" or "nearly every day"). Thus, the PHQ-15 score ranges from 0 to 30; cutpoints of 5, 10, and 15 represent mild, moderate, and severe somatization, respectively. The PHQ-15 also has two component scores: the 5 pain items that produce a somatic pain score that ranges from 0 to 10, and the other 10 items that produce a somatic nonpain score that ranges from 0 to 20. There is good evidence that the PHQ-9 is sensitive to change when used for monitoring outcomes in the treatment of depression [77], whereas preliminary evidence for the responsiveness of the PHQ-15 [78] requires further validation in clinical trials. Regarding anxiety, the original PHQ is good for establishing diagnoses of panic disorder and has a general scale for "other anxiety disorder." Also, a 7-item PHQ measure for generalized anxiety disorder has recently been developed (Spitzer et al, unpublished data) [79].

Managing symptoms

Management can be divided into two phases: the initial approach to the symptomatic patient, and follow-up care for those with persistent symptoms. Described in detail elsewhere [1,2,63], the core components of a stepped care approach are summarized in Table 2.

Initial visit

A conservative approach is warranted initially because 75% or more of patients improve within 2 to 6 weeks, regardless of the type of symptom. Thus, a brief, focused evaluation with follow-up, rather than an exhaustive work-up, is appropriate for most patients who have physical symptoms. For some symptoms (eg, dizziness, back pain, chronic cough), research supports a brief office examination that focuses on a few key elements of the history and physical examination [80–82]. More evidence-based algorithms that allow efficient evaluation of common symptoms are needed. Some symptoms (eg, angina-like chest pain, dyspnea with an abnormal cardiopulmonary examination, acute abdominal pain, syncope) require a lower threshold for a comprehensive initial workup, whereas other symptoms seldom are acutely serious (eg, back pain, fatigue, insomnia). Although "red flags" on history or physical examination can trigger an expedited work-up for any symptom, it is estimated that the minority ($<5\%$) of physical symptoms that are seen in primary care office practice are acutely serious [2].

Although symptoms are ubiquitous, only a small proportion of individuals seek health care for their complaints [83–85]. In short, only a minority of symptomatic persons become true patients [86]. Although this can be prompted by symptom severity or persistence, many individuals come to the clinic because of symptom-related concerns and expectations [87–89]. Serious illness worry—either disease-specific (Could this headache be a brain tumor?) or generic (I don't know what this might be, but is it something to worry about?)—is one of the most common concerns. Prognosis is another frequent concern (eg, How long is this likely to last? Will it interfere with my work or recreational activities?). Common expectations for

Table 2
Approach to the patient who has unexplained physical symptoms

Action	Examples
Initial Visit	
Symptom-specific evaluation	Evidence-based interview and physical examination
	Some symptom patterns can be worrisome (eg, angina-like chest pain; dyspnea with abnormal lung auscultation; acute abdominal pain; syncope)
	Other symptoms are serious in only a small minority of patients (back pain, fatigue, insomnia)
	Look for "red flags" (eg, focal neurologic findings in patient who has dizziness or headache; hypotension or abnormal cardiac examination in patient who has syncope)
Address symptom-specific concerns and expectations	"Is there anything else you were worried about?" (serious cause? How long symptom might last?)
	"Is there anything else you wanted or thought might be helpful? (test? referral? treatment?)
Generic symptom treatment	Analgesics for pain. Gastrointestinal medications for dyspepsia or constipation.
Watchful waiting	Have patient follow-up in 2–6 wk if symptom not resolved
Follow-up visits	
Psychologic screening	Especially screen for potentially treatable depressive and anxiety disorders. Assess somatization.
Diagnostic evaluation	Selective diagnostic testing or specialty referral, especially if new unexplained symptom, if findings on interview or examination are worrisome for serious cause, or if patient insists
Chronic symptom therapies	Pharmacologic: analgesics, gastrointestinal medications, antidepressants
	Nonpharmacologic: cognitive-behavioral therapy, other behavioral therapies, exercise, pain self-management programs, reattribution
Strategies in managing chronic somatization	Schedule regular, brief appointments that are not related to symptom exacerbations
	Avoid diagnostic tests and subspecialty referral, especially for symptoms that were evaluated previously
	When new symptoms arise, conduct focused evaluations and testing rather than exhaustive work-ups
	Empathize with the complaint. Do not dispute the reality of the symptom or associated impairment.
	Focus on symptom management/reduction rather than elimination (coping rather than cure)
	Strive for rehabilitation (maximizing function despite the symptom) rather than disability
	Emphasize that referral is for consultation or comanagement rather than dismissal ("dumping")

provider actions include medication prescriptions, diagnostic tests, or sub-specialty referrals. Patients frequently do not reveal their concerns and expectations unless specifically invited to do so, and clinicians often fail to elicit them. Patients may be reluctant to volunteer their "hidden agenda" because of embarrassment (Are my concerns foolish or unreasonable?), fear of wasting the doctor's time, or the mistaken assumption that if it is important, the doctor will ask. Addressing the patient's concerns and expectations can improve patient and provider satisfaction, adherence with the physician's recommendations, and possibly, symptom outcome [90–92]. Two useful questions to ask at the end of the initial visit are "Is there anything else that you were worried about?" and "Is there anything else that you wanted or thought might be helpful?".

Symptomatic treatment if available (eg, analgesics for pain, gastrointestinal medications for dyspepsia or bowel complaints) and advising the patient to follow-up if the symptom does not improve within 2 to 4 weeks is a reasonable strategy in many cases.

Follow-up for persistent symptoms

Psychologic screening for potentially treatable depressive, anxiety, and somatoform disorders is indicated in persons who have persistent symptoms. Also, physical or sexual abuse increases the risk for unexplained symptoms, as do other types of trauma or violence. Selective diagnostic testing or specialty referral may be considered, especially if this is a new unexplained symptom, if findings on interview or examination are worrisome for a serious cause, or if the patient is insistent on further evaluation. Pharmacologic therapies, such as analgesics and gastrointestinal medications, are available for certain chronic symptoms. Antidepressants may be a useful adjunct therapy in a variety of symptom syndromes, including migraine and tension headache, fibromyalgia, irritable bowel syndrome, tinnitus, and chronic pain [93,94]. Likewise, cognitive behavioral therapy has well-established efficacy for these same conditions as well as back pain and chronic fatigue syndrome [94,95]. Other types of behavioral therapy also may be beneficial for certain symptoms [96,97]. Reattribution is another approach that is useful in patients who have somatized mental disorder [98]. Exercise programs can reduce symptoms in chronic fatigue syndrome, fibromyalgia, and back pain. Also, pain self-management programs are beneficial [99,100]. Selected strategies for patients who have chronic somatization are highlighted in Table 2, with the topic reviewed more thoroughly elsewhere [101].

More advanced strategies can be helpful in complicated patients. Improved training of nonpsychiatric physicians in skills that can be incorporated efficiently into clinical practice (eg, The Extended Reattribution and Management [TERM] model) is beneficial and, if implemented broadly, might be one approach to improving outcomes in larger numbers of somatizing patients [102]. In the patient who has more chronic or severe symptoms, an integrated risk assessment that looks for different foci of intervention, such as with the INTERMED (see the article by Stiefel and colleagues elsewhere in this issue) might be appropriate. Other patients are sufficiently complex that treatment should proceed directly toward case management [103].

No area of medicine requires tearing down the walls of mind–body dualism more than the interface between somatic and psychologic symptoms. Integrating medical and psychiatric care is essential to the patient-centered and cost-effective care of symptoms. Leigh Hunt, a nineteenth century poet recognized: "The mind may undoubtedly affect the body; but the body also affects the mind. There is a re-action between them; and by lessening it on either side, you diminish the pain on both."

References

[1] Kroenke K. Studying symptoms: sampling and measurement issues. Ann Intern Med 2001; 134:844–55.
[2] Kroenke K. Patients presenting with somatic complaints: epidemiology, psychiatric comorbidity and management. Int J Methods Psychiatr Res 2003;12:34–43.
[3] Kroenke K, Jackson JL. Outcome in general medical patients presenting with common symptoms: a prospective study with a 2-week and a 3-month follow-up. Fam Pract 1998; 15:398–403.
[4] Jackson JL, Passamonti ML. the outcomes among patients presenting in primary care with a physical symptoms at 5 years. J Gen Intern Med 2005;20:1032–7.
[5] Kroenke K, Lucas CA, Rosenberg ML, et al. Causes of persistent dizziness: a prospective study of 100 patients in ambulatory care. Ann Intern Med 1992;117:898–904.
[6] Celentano DD, Stewart WF, Linet MS. The relationship of headache symptoms with severity and duration of attacks. J Clin Epidemiol 1990;43:983–94.
[7] Von Korff MR, Howard JA, Truelove EL, et al. Temporomandibular disorders. Variation in clinical practice. Med Care 1988;26:307–14.
[8] Jensen MC, Brant-Zawadzki MN, Obuchowski N, et al. Magnetic resonance imaging of the lumbar spine in people without back pain. N Engl J Med 1994;331:69–73.
[9] Donovan LE, Corenblum B. The natural history of the pituitary incidentaloma. Arch Intern Med 1995;155:181–3.
[10] Tan GH, Gharib H. Thyroid incidentalomas: management approaches to nonpalpable nodules discovered incidentally on thyroid imaging. Ann Intern Med 1997;126:226–31.
[11] Sigal LH. The Lyme disease controversy. Social and financial costs of misdiagnosis and mismanagement. Arch Intern Med 1996;156:1493–500.
[12] Steere AC, Taylor E, McHugh GL, et al. The overdiagnosis of Lyme disease. JAMA 1993; 269:1812–6.
[13] Meador CK. The art and science of nondisease. N Engl J Med 1965;272:92–5.
[14] Kroenke K, Wood DR, Mangelsdorff AD, et al. Chronic fatigue in primary care: prevalence, patient characteristics, and outcome. JAMA 1988;260:929–34.
[15] Kroenke K, Lucas C, Rosenberg ML, et al. One-year outcome in patients with a chief complaint of dizziness. J Gen Intern Med 1994;9:684–9.
[16] Martina B, Bucheli B, Stotz M, et al. First clinical judgment by primary care physicians distinguishes well between nonorganic and organic causes of abdominal or chest pain. J Gen Intern Med 1997;12:459–65.
[17] Wasson JH, Sox HC Jr, Sox CH. The diagnosis of abdominal pain in ambulatory male patients. Med Decis Making 1981;1:215–24.
[18] Sox HC, Margulies I, Sox CH. Psychologically mediated effects of diagnostic tests. Ann Intern Med 1981;95:680–5.

[19] Weber BE, Kapoor WN. Evaluation and outcomes of patients with palpitations. Am J Med 1996;100:138–48.
[20] Von Korff M, Deyo RA, Cherkin D, et al. Back pain in primary care. Outcomes at 1 year. Spine 1993;18:855–62.
[21] Martin RD. The somatoform conundrum: a question of nosological values. Gen Hosp Psychiatry 1999;21:177–86.
[22] Mayou R, Kirmayer LJ, Simon G, et al. Somatoform disorders: time for a new approach in DSM-V. Am J Psychiatry 2005;162:847–55.
[23] Clark LA, Livesley WJ, Morey L. Personality disorder assessment: the challenge of construct validity. J Personal Disord 1997;11:205–31.
[24] Widiger TA, Clark LA. Toward DSM-V and the classification of psychopathology. Psychol Bull 2000;126:946–63.
[25] Escobar JI, Gara M, Silver RC, et al. Somatisation disorder in primary care. Br J Psychiatry 1998;173:262–6.
[26] Katon W, Lin E, Von Korff M, et al. Somatization: a spectrum of severity. Am J Psychiatry 1991;148:34–40.
[27] Kirmayer LJ, Robbins JM. Three forms of somatization in primary care: prevalence, co-occurrence, and sociodemographic characteristics. J Nerv Ment Dis 1991;179:647–55.
[28] Spitzer RL, Wakefield JC. DSM-IV diagnostic criterion for clinical significance: does it help solve the false positives problem? Am J Psychiatry 1999;156:1856–64.
[29] de Waal MW, Arnold IA, Eekhof JA, et al. Somatoform disorders in general practice: prevalence, functional impairment and comorbidity with anxiety and depressive disorders. Br J Psychiatry 2004;184:470–6.
[30] Kroenke K, Spitzer RL, deGruy FV, et al. Multisomatoform disorder: an alternative to undifferentiated somatoform disorder for the somatizing patient in primary care. Arch Gen Psychiatry 1997;54:352–8.
[31] Noyes R Jr. The relationship of hypochondriasis to anxiety disorders. Gen Hosp Psychiatry 1999;21:8–17.
[32] Phillips KA, McElroy SL, Hudson JI, et al. Body dysmorphic disorder: an obsessive-compulsive spectrum disorder, a form of affective spectrum disorder, or both? J Clin Psychiatry 1995;56(Suppl 4):41–51.
[33] Bass C, Murphy M. Somatoform and personality disorders: syndromal comorbidity and overlapping developmental pathways. J Psychosom Res 1995;39:403–27.
[34] Birket-Smith M, Mortensen EL. Pain in somatoform disorders: is somatoform pain disorder a valid diagnosis? Acta Psychiatr Scand 2002;106:103–8.
[35] Kessler RC, McGonagle KA, Zhao S, et al. Lifetime and 12-month prevalence of DSM-III-R psychiatric disorders in the United States: results from the National Comorbidity Survey. Arch Gen Psychiatry 1994;51:8–19.
[36] Bijl RV, Ravelli A, van Zessen G. Prevalence of psychiatric disorder in the general population: results of The Netherlands Mental Health Survey and Incidence Study (NEMESIS). Soc Psychiatry Psychiatr Epidemiol 1998;33:587–95.
[37] Oldham JM, Skodol AE, Kellman HD, et al. Diagnosis of DSM-III-R personality disorders by two structured interviews: patterns of comorbidity. Am J Psychiatry 1992;149:213–20.
[38] Zimmerman M, Coryell W. DSM-III personality disorder diagnoses in a nonpatient sample. Demographic correlates and comorbidity. Arch Gen Psychiatry 1989;46:682–9.
[39] McGlashan TH, Grilo CM, Skodol AE, et al. The Collaborative Longitudinal Personality Disorders Study: baseline Axis I/II and II/II diagnostic co-occurrence. Acta Psychiatr Scand 2000;102:256–64.
[40] Ormel J, Vonkorff M, Ustun TB, et al. Common mental disorders and disability across cultures. Results from the WHO Collaborative Study on Psychological Problems in General Health Care. JAMA 1994;272:1741–8.

[41] Brown FW, Golding JM, Smith GR. Psychiatric comorbidity in primary care somatization disorder. Psychosom Med 1990;52:445–51.

[42] Rost KM, Akins RN, Brown FW, et al. The comorbidity of DSM-III-R personality disorders in somatization disorder. Gen Hosp Psychiatry 1992;14:322–6.

[43] Wessely S, Nimnuan C, Sharpe M. Functional somatic syndromes: one or many? Lancet 1999;354:936–9.

[44] Barsky AJ, Borus JF. Functional somatic syndromes. Ann Intern Med 1999;130:910–21.

[45] Aaron LA, Buchwald D. A review of the evidence for overlap among unexplained clinical conditions. Ann Intern Med 2001;134:868–81.

[46] Light RW, Merrill EJ, Despars J, et al. Doxepin treatment of depressed patients with chronic obstructive pulmonary disease. Arch Intern Med 1986;146:1377–80.

[47] Lustman PJ, Clouse RE, Carney RM. Depression and the reporting of diabetes symptoms. Int J Psychiatry Med 1988;18:295–303.

[48] Ludman EJ, Katon W, Russo J, et al. Depression and diabetes symptom burden. Gen Hosp Psychiatry 2004;26:430–6.

[49] Barsky AJ, Ahern DK, Bailey D, et al. Predictors of persistent palpitations and continued medical utilization. J Fam Pract 1996;42:465–72.

[50] Ruo B, Rumsfeld JS, Hlatky MA, et al. Depressive symptoms and health-related quality of life: the Heart and Soul Study. JAMA 2003;290:215–21.

[51] Vingerhoets G, De Soete G, Jannes C. Subjective complaints versus neuropsychological test performance after cardiopulmonary bypass. J Psychosom Res 1995;39:843–53.

[52] Novy D, Berry MP, Palmer JL, et al. Somatic symptoms in patients with chronic non-cancer-related and cancer-related pain. J Pain Symptom Manage 2005;29:603–12.

[53] Kilbourne AM, Justice AC, Rollman BL, et al. Clinical importance of HIV and depressive symptoms among veterans with HIV infection. J Gen Intern Med 2002;17:512–20.

[54] Sha MC, Callahan CM, Counsell SR, et al. Physical symptoms as a predictor of health care use and mortality among older adults. Am J Med 2005;118:301–6.

[55] Wagstaff AJ, Cheer SM, Matheson AJ, et al. Spotlight on paroxetine in psychiatric disorders in adults. CNS Drugs 2002;16:425–34.

[56] Silver H. Selective serotonin re-uptake inhibitor augmentation in the treatment of negative symptoms of schizophrenia. Expert Opin Pharmacother 2004;5:2053–8.

[57] Fountoulakis KN, Nimatoudis I, Iacovides A, et al. Off-label indications for atypical antipsychotics: a systematic review. Ann Gen Hosp Psychiatry 2004;3:4.

[58] Katon W, Kleinman A, Rosen G. Depression and somatization: a review. Part I. Am J Med 1982;72:127–35.

[59] Kroenke K, Spitzer RL, Williams JBW, et al. Physical symptoms in primary care: predictors of psychiatric disorders and functional impairment. Arch Fam Med 1994;3:774–9.

[60] Kroenke K, Jackson JL, Chamberlin J. Depressive and anxiety disorders in patients presenting with physical complaints: clinical predictors and outcome. Am J Med 1997;103: 339–47.

[61] Simon G, Gater R, Kisely S, Piccinelli M. Somatic symptoms of distress: an international primary care study. Psychosom Med 1996;58:481–8.

[62] Simon GE, Von Korff M. Somatization and psychiatric disorder in the NIMH Epidemiologic Catchment Area study. Am J Psychiatry 1991;148:1494–500.

[63] Kroenke K. The interface between physical and psychological symptoms. Prim Care Companion J Clin Psychiatry 2003;5(Suppl 7):11–8.

[64] Reid S, Wessely S, Crayford T, et al. Medically unexplained symptoms in frequent attenders of secondary health care: retrospective cohort study. BMJ 2001;322:1–4.

[65] Henningsen P, Zimmermann T, Sattel H. Medically unexplained physical symptoms, anxiety, and depression: a meta-analytic review. Psychosom Med 2003;65:528–33.

[66] Hahn SR. Physical symptoms and physician-experienced difficulty in the physician-patient relationship. Ann Intern Med 2001;134:897–904.

[67] Hahn SR, Kroenke K, Spitzer RL, et al. The difficult patient: prevalence, psychopathology, and functional impairment. J Gen Intern Med 1996;11:1–8.
[68] Jackson JL, Kroenke K. Difficult patient encounters in the ambulatory clinic: clinical predictors and outcomes. Arch Intern Med 1999;159:1069–75.
[69] Katon W, Sullivan M, Walker E. Medical symptoms without identified pathology: relationship to psychiatric disorders, childhood and adult trauma, and personality traits. Ann Intern Med 2001;134:917–25.
[70] Barsky AJ, Saintfort R, Rogers MP, et al. Nonspecific medication side effects and the nocebo phenomenon. JAMA 2002;287:622–7.
[71] Williams JWJ, Noel PH, Cordes JA, et al. Is this patient clinically depressed? JAMA 2002;287:1160–70.
[72] Spitzer RL, Kroenke K, Williams JBW, the Patient Health Questionnaire Study Group. Validity and utility of a self-report version of PRIME-MD: The PHQ Primary Care Study. JAMA 1999;282:1737–44.
[73] Spitzer RL, Williams JBW, Kroenke K, et al. Validity and utility of the Patient Health Questionnaire in assessment of 3000 obstetric-gynecologic patients: the PRIME-MD Patient Health Questionnaire Obstetrics-Gynecology Study. Am J Obstet Gynecol 2000;183:759–69.
[74] Kroenke K, Spitzer RL. The PHQ-9: A new depression and diagnostic severity measure. Psychiatr Ann 2002;32:509–21.
[75] Kroenke K, Spitzer RL, Williams JBW. The PHQ-9: validity of a brief depression severity measure. J Gen Intern Med 2001;16:606–13.
[76] Kroenke K, Spitzer RL, Williams JBW. The PHQ-15: validity of a new measure for evaluating the severity of somatic symptoms. Psychosom Med 2001;64:258–66.
[77] Lowe B, Unutzer J, Callahan CM. et al. Monitoring depression treatment outcomes with the patient health questionnaire-9. Med Care 2004;42:1194–201.
[78] Kroenke K, Messina N, Benattia I, et al. Venlafaxine extended-release in the short-term treatment of depressed and anxious primary care patients with multisomatoform disorder. J Clin Psychiatry 2006;67(1):72–80.
[79] Spitzer RL, Kroenke K, Williams JBW, et al. A brief measure for assessing generalized anxiety disorder: the GAD-7. Arch Intern Med 2006;166:1092–7.
[80] Kroenke K, Hoffman RM, Einstadter D. A rational approach to the dizzy patient. Journal of Clinical Outcomes Management 1997;4:33–41.
[81] Atlas SJ, Deyo RA. Evaluating and managing acute low back pain in the primary care setting. J Gen Intern Med 2001;16:120–31.
[82] Irwin RS, Madison JM. Symptom research on chronic cough: a historical perspective. Ann Intern Med 2001;134:809–14.
[83] Banks MH, Beresford SA, Morrell DC, et al. Factors influencing demand for primary medical care in women aged 20–44 years: a preliminary report. Int J Epidemiol 1975;4:189–95.
[84] Verbrugge LM, Ascione FJ. Exploring the iceberg: common symptoms and how people care for them. Med Care 1987;25:539–69.
[85] Green LA, Fryer GE, Yawn BP, et al. The ecology of medical care revisited. N Engl J Med 2001;344:2021–5.
[86] Eisenberg L. What makes persons "patients" and patients "well"?. Am J Med 1980;69:277–86.
[87] Kravitz RL, Callahan EJ, Paterniti D, et al. Prevalence and sources of patients' unmet expectations for care. Ann Intern Med 1996;125:730–7.
[88] Jackson JL, Kroenke K. The effect of unmet expectations among adults presenting with physical symptoms. Ann Intern Med 2001;134:889–97.
[89] Bell RA, Kravitz RL, Thom D, et al. Unmet expectations for care and the patient-physician relationship. J Gen Intern Med 2002;17:817–24.

[90] Jackson JL, Kroenke K, Chamberlin J. Effects of physician awareness of symptom-related expectations and mental disorders: a controlled trial. Arch Fam Med 1999;8:135–42.

[91] Hornberger J, Thom D, MaCurdy T. Effects of a self-administered previsit questionnaire to enhance awareness of patients' concerns in primary care. J Gen Intern Med 1997;12: 597–606.

[92] Bell RA, Kravitz RL, Thom D, et al. Unsaid but not forgotten: patients' unvoiced desires in office visits. Arch Intern Med 2001;161:1977–84.

[93] O'Malley PG, Jackson JL, Santoro J, et al. Antidepressant therapy for unexplained symptoms and symptom syndromes. J Fam Pract 1999;48:980–90.

[94] Jackson JL, O'Malley PG, Kroenke K. Antidepressants and cognitive behavioral therapy for symptom syndromes. CNS Spectr 2006;11:212–22.

[95] Kroenke K, Swindle R. Cognitive-behavioral therapy for somatization and symptom syndromes: a critical review of controlled clinical trials. Psychother Psychosom 2000;69: 205–15.

[96] Allen LA, Escobar JI, Lehrer PM, et al. Psychosocial treatments for multiple unexplained physical symptoms: a review of the literature. Psychosom Med 2002;64:939–50.

[97] Raine R, Haines A, Sensky T, et al. Systematic review of mental health interventions for patients with common somatic symptoms: can research evidence from secondary care be extrapolated to primary care? BMJ 2002;325:1082.

[98] Morriss RK, Gask L. Treatment of patients with somatized mental disorder: effects of re-attribution training on outcomes under the direct control of the family doctor. Psychosomatics 2002;43:394–9.

[99] Lorig KR, Holman H. Self-management education: history, definition, outcomes, and mechanisms. Ann Behav Med 2003;26:1–7.

[100] Damush TM, Weinberger M, Perkins SM, et al. Randomized trial of a self-management program for primary care patients with acute low back pain: short-term effects. Arthritis Rheum 2003;49:179–86.

[101] Smith RC, Lein C, Collins C, et al. Treating patients with medically unexplained symptoms in primary care. J Gen Intern Med 2003;18:478–89.

[102] Fink P, Rosendal M, Toft T. Assessment and treatment of functional disorders in general practice: the extended reattribution and management model—an advanced educational program for nonpsychiatric doctors. Psychosomatics 2002;43:93–131.

[103] Smith RC, Lyles JS, Gardiner JC, et al. Primary care clinicians treat patients with medically unexplained symptoms—a randomized controlled trial. J Gen Intern Med 2006;21:671–7.

ELSEVIER
SAUNDERS

Med Clin N Am 90 (2006) 627–646

THE MEDICAL
CLINICS
OF NORTH AMERICA

Disease-Focused or Integrated Treatment: Diabetes and Depression

Leonard E. Egede, MD, MS[a,b],*

[a]Medical University of South Carolina, Center for Health Disparities Research,
135 Rutledge Avenue, Room 280H, PO Box 250593, Charleston, SC 29425, USA
[b]Charleston VA Targeted Research Enhancement Program, Ralph H. Johnson VAMC,
Charleston, SC, USA

Worldwide burden of diabetes

The prevalence of diabetes mellitus is approaching epidemic proportions across the world. In the United States, current estimates indicate that 7.0% of the population or 20.8 million people have diabetes. Of this number, 14.6 million are diagnosed cases, whereas 6.2 million are undiagnosed. Based on 2005 data, the incidence of diabetes in the United States is approximately 1.5 million cases per year. These numbers represent a significant increase from previous years. For example, the age-adjusted incidence of diagnosed diabetes increased from 2.77% in 1980 to 4.22% in 1999 and the incidence of diabetes increased from 0.23% in 1980 to 0.34% in 1999. Diabetes is the leading cause of cardiovascular disease, strokes, blindness, and lower limb amputations. It was the sixth leading cause of death listed on U.S. death certificates in 2002, and individuals who have diabetes have a twofold increased risk for death compared with individuals who do not have diabetes of similar age and sex. Diabetes also is associated with increased health care costs. In 2002, the total cost of diabetes in the United States was $132 billion. Of this amount, $92 billion was from the direct medical cost of diabetes, whereas $40 billion was from disability, work loss, and premature mortality [1,2].

Diabetes also is a major problem in other parts of the world. Available data indicate that in 1995, 4.0% of the world population or 135 million people had diabetes. This number is expected to increase to 300 million or 5.4%

Dr. Egede is supported in part by Grant No. 5K08HS11418 from the Agency for Healthcare Research and Quality.

* Center for Health Disparities Research, Medical University of South Carolina, 135 Rutledge Avenue, Suite 280H, Charleston, SC 29425.

E-mail address: egedel@musc.edu

of the world population by the year 2025. It is projected that by 2025, the prevalence of diabetes will increase by 42% in the developed world and by 170% in the developing world. The projections also suggest that by 2025, more than 75% of the world population with diabetes will reside in developing countries and that the individual countries with the largest population of adults who have diabetes will include India, China, and the United States [3].

Worldwide burden of depression

Depression is another disease that is highly prevalent in most countries of the world. In the United States, depression affects 9.5% of the adult population or 19 million people in any given year [4], and women have a twofold higher prevalence of depression compared with men (W.E. Narrow, unpublished data) [5]. A recent study in the United States found that the lifetime prevalence of major depressive disorder was 16.2%, whereas the 12-month prevalence was 6.6% [6]. A recent study from Europe found that 14% of European adults have a lifetime prevalence of a mood disorder and 4.2% have a 12-month prevalence of a mood disorder [7]. Another study was conducted recently to determine the prevalence of mood disorders in 14 countries in the Americas, Europe, the Middle East, Africa, and Asia [8]. The 12-month prevalence of mood disorders was 0.8% in Nigeria, 3.1% in Japan, 6.6% in Lebanon, 6.8% in Columbia, 6.9% in the Netherlands, 8.5% in France, 9.1% in the Ukraine, and 9.6% in the United States. Major depression is the second leading cause of disability-adjusted life years (DALYs) lost in women and the tenth leading cause of DALYs in men [9]. Studies also showed that depression is a major contributor to work place absenteeism, diminished or lost productivity, and increased use of health services [10].

Prevalence of depression in individuals who have diabetes

The observation that there is a relationship between diabetes and depression was made first in 1684 by Dr. Thomas Willis, a British physician who suggested that diabetes resulted from "sadness or long sorrow" [11]. Studies that were conducted in the 1980s found that there was an increased prevalence of depression in persons who had diabetes [12–14]. In 1993, Gavard and colleagues [15] reviewed 20 published studies on the association between diabetes and depression. They found that the prevalence of depression in individuals who had diabetes ranged from 8.5% (studies based on diagnostic instruments) to 27.3% (studies based on self-report instruments). Anderson and colleagues [16] conducted a meta-analysis of 42 published studies that included 21,351 adults. They found that the prevalence of major depression in people who had diabetes was 11% and the prevalence of clinically relevant depression was 31%. Two recent studies used data that were representative of the U.S. population to estimate the likelihood of depression and the prevalence of major depression in adults who had diabetes [17,18]. The first study found that adults who had diabetes were twice as likely to have depression compared with adults who did not have diabetes [17]. Using a diagnostic instrument, the second study found that the prevalence of major depressive disorder in adults who had diabetes was 9.3% compared with 6.1% in adults who did not have diabetes [18]. Overall, these studies have shown consistently that individuals who have diabetes are more likely to have depression than are individuals who do not have diabetes.

Effect of depression on glycemic control and risk for diabetes complications

There is overwhelming evidence that the coexistence of diabetes and depression is associated with poor diabetes outcomes. In a large meta-analysis that included individuals who had type 1 and type 2 diabetes, depression was associated significantly with poor glycemic control [19]. The standardized effect size (ES) was in the small to moderate range (0.17) and was consistent (95% CI, 0.13–0.21). ESs were similar for type 1 and type 2 diabetes, but were larger when diagnostic criteria rather than self-report questionnaires were used to assess depression (0.28 versus 0.15, respectively). Depression also increases the odds of having diabetes complications. In another meta-analysis, comorbid depression was associated significantly with a variety of diabetes complications, including retinopathy, nephropathy, neuropathy, macrovascular complications, and sexual dysfunction [20]. In that study, ESs were in the small to moderate range (ES, 0.17–0.32). In the Hispanic Established Population for the Epidemiologic Study of the Elderly (EPESE) Survey, comorbid depression was associated significantly with an increased risk for macro- and microvascular complications in elderly Mexican Americans who had type 2 diabetes [21].

Effect of depression on disability, work productivity, and quality of life

Several studies showed that comorbid depression is associated with decreased function and increased odds of lost productivity. In the Hispanic EPESE survey, the coexistence of diabetes and depression was associated with an increased risk for disability among older Mexican Americans [21]. In that study, patients who had diabetes and coexisting depression had a 4.1-fold increased odds for disability, whereas those who had diabetes or depression alone had a 1.7-fold and a 1.3-fold increased odds for disability, respectively. In another study, data on 30,022 adults from a representative sample of the U.S. population were analyzed to determine the effect of depression on functional disability in adults with diabetes [22]. In that study, the odds of functional disability were 3.00 (95% CI, 2.62–3.42) for adults who had major depression, 2.42 (95% CI, 2.10–2.79) for those who had diabetes, and 7.15 (95% CI, 4.53–11.28) for those who had diabetes and depression. These studies show that the coexistence of diabetes and major depression has a synergistic effect on the odds of disability. Another study assessed the effect of major depression on lost productivity in adults who had diabetes [23]. Individuals who had diabetes and coexisting depression missed more days from work, spent more days in bed because of disability, and were more likely to miss at least 7 days of work in any given year. In a study of 3010 Australian adults, the coexistence of diabetes and depression was associated with significantly lower physical and mental health component scores of the Medical Outcomes Survey Short Form-36 scale compared with those who had diabetes or depression alone [24].

Effect of depression on health care costs

Several studies showed that comorbid depression is associated with increased health care costs in patients who have diabetes. A study of 367 subjects who had diabetes found that people who had depression had almost a twofold increase in health care cost compared with people who did not have depression (unadjusted 6-month total health care cost $3654 versus $2094) [25]. In another study of 825 subjects who had diabetes, the U.S. population–weighted health care cost was 4.5-fold higher in people who had depression compared with those who did not have depression ($247 million versus $55 million) [17]. Another study analyzed Medicare claims data in elderly subjects who had diabetes and found that those who had depression had a twofold increased health care cost compared with those who did not have depression ($25,360 versus $10,358) [26]. A more recent study used claims data to calculate the 3-year health care cost in 1694 adults who had diabetes [27]. Standardized costs for those who had depression were significantly higher than the costs for those who did not have depression ($31,967 versus $21,609). These studies confirm that comorbid depression is associated with increased health care costs in people who have diabetes

Effect of depression on medication adherence

Diabetes is a complex and progressive metabolic disease that requires treatment with multiple medications. Medication adherence is critical to achieving metabolic control in diabetes. Several studies in persons who had diabetes showed a high correlation between medication adherence and metabolic control. A study of 301 subjects who had type 2 diabetes assessed the relationship between medication adherence by a validated self-report questionnaire and hemoglobin A1C (HbA_{1c}) levels [28]. Good adherence was associated with a 10% lower HbA_{1c} level after adjusting for important confounding variables, including age, gender, race/ethnicity, duration of disease, presence of complications, and practice factors. In another study of 810 patients who had type 2 diabetes and were on oral diabetes medications, the association between HbA_{1c} level as well as change in HbA_{1c} level with medication adherence (using prescription refill data) were assessed [29]. Better metabolic control was associated independently with greater medication adherence; each 10% increment in medication adherence resulted in a 0.16% decrease in HbA_{1c} after controlling for demographic and clinical characteristics.

Other studies that used objective measures of medication adherence, including pill counts [30,31] and pharmacy records [32], demonstrated similar associations between medication adherence and metabolic control in persons who had type 2 diabetes; however, a recent systematic review of medication adherence in persons who had diabetes found that many patients for whom diabetic medications were prescribed adhered to treatment poorly [33]. In that review, retrospective analyses showed that adherence to oral diabetic medications ranged from 36% to 93%, whereas prospective electronic monitoring showed that adherence ranged from 67% to 85%.

Depression is known to be a major barrier to medication adherence in patients who have medical conditions. Recently, a meta-analysis was conducted to assess the effect of depression on medication adherence and adherence to health behavior regimens in patients who had medical conditions [34]. This study analyzed data from 12 published studies with a total sample size of 661 subjects. Patients who had comorbid depression were three times more likely to be nonadherent to medical treatment compared with patients who did not have depression. In another study that included 367 subjects who had diabetes, depressed patients spent more days without oral hypoglycemic medications compared with those who were not depressed (14.9 versus 7.1 days) [25]. Another study examined the effect of depression on medication adherence in 4463 subjects who had diabetes and found that depressed patients had more days of nonadherence to oral hypoglycemic medications than did nondepressed patients (80 versus 62 days) [35]. A more recent study of 203 patients who had diabetes found that those who had depression had fewer days with adequate medication coverage than did those who did not have depression [36]. Thus, the coexistence of diabetes and depression is associated with significantly increased odds of medication nonadherence in patients who have diabetes.

Effect of depression on diabetes self-care behaviors

Adoption of appropriate self-care behaviors is an integral part of good diabetes care. Evidence from large clinical trials showed that regular exercise training, appropriate dietary intake, and daily monitoring of home blood glucose are necessary to achieve glycemic, lipid, and blood pressure control in people who have diabetes [37]. Several studies showed that few patients who have diabetes meet recommended guidelines for physical activity, dietary intake, or self-monitoring of blood glucose [38–40]. The already low adherence to self-care recommendations in people who have diabetes is worsened by coexisting depression. Multiple studies showed that in addition to other psychosocial barriers to guideline adherence, depression is a major reason for nonadherence to health behavior recommendations in people who have diabetes [25,35,41]. Table 1 shows the association of depression with diabetes self-care behaviors.

Effect of depression on mortality

Four recent studies found that coexisting depression increased the risk for death in people who had diabetes [21,42–44]. In the Hispanic EPESE Survey, 2830 Mexican Americans aged 65 years or older were assessed for depression at baseline and followed for more than 7 years. The interaction of diabetes and depression was synergistic and predicted greater mortality even after controlling for sociodemographic characteristics and marital status [21]. Interaction of diabetes and depression was associated with a four-fold increased risk for death (Odds Ratio, 4.04; 95% CI, 2.70–6.02). Another study analyzed longitudinal data from the first National Health and Nutrition Examination Survey (NHANES) I Epidemiologic Follow-up Study and found that diabetic persons with Center for Epidemiology Study Depression Scale scores of at least 16 had a 54% greater mortality than did those with scores of less than 16 [42]. In another study, 10,025 participants in the population-based NHANES I Epidemiologic Follow-up Study were followed for more than 8 years to evaluate the effect of depression on all-cause and coronary heart disease (CHD) mortality among adults who did and did not have diabetes (Fig. 1) [43]. Hazard rates of death for people who had diabetes and depression were 2.50 (95% CI, 2.04–3.08) for all-cause mortality and 2.43 (95% CI, 1.66–3.56) for CHD mortality. The most recent study was conducted on 4154 patients who had type 2

Table 1
Relationship of depression and diabetes self-care behaviors

Self-care activities (past 7 days)	Major depression	No major depression	Odds ratio	95% CI
Healthy eating once weekly or less	17.2%	8.8%	2.1	1.59–2.72
5 servings of fruits and vegetables once weekly or less	32.4%	21.1%	1.8	1.43–2.17
High-fat foods ≥6 times weekly	15.5%	11.9%	1.3	1.01–1.73
Physical activity (≥30 min) once weekly or less	44.1%	27.3%	1.9	1.53–2.27
Specific exercise session once weekly or less	62.1%	45.8%	1.7	1.43–2.12
Smoking: yes	16.1%	7.7%	1.9	1.42–2.51

Adapted from Lin EH, Katon W, Von Korff M, et al. Relationship of depression and diabetes self-care, medication adherence, and preventive care. Diabetes Care 2004;27(9):2157.

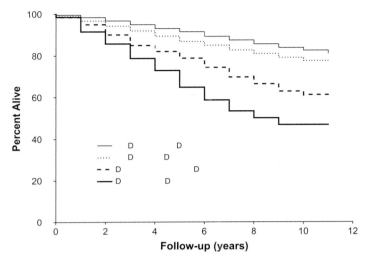

Fig. 1. Effect of depression on all-cause mortality in patients who have diabetes. (*Adapted from* Egede LE, Nietert PJ, Zheng D. Depression and all-cause and coronary heart disease mortality among adults with and without diabetes. Diabetes Care 2005;28(6):1342; with permission).

diabetes who were followed for up to 3 years [44]. Compared with the non-depressed group, those who had minor depression had a 1.67-fold increased risk for death, whereas those who had major depression had a 2.30-fold increased risk for death over the 3-year period.

Causal pathways between diabetes and depression

There are two major hypotheses about the causal pathways between diabetes and depression (also see the article by Gans elsewhere in this issue). One hypothesis is that depression precedes type 2 diabetes (ie, depression increases the risk for developing diabetes). Data from several studies are supportive of this hypothesis [45–48]; however, this association has not been consistent across studies, and some studies found no significant association between depression and the increased risk for developing diabetes [49–51]. The underlying mechanism for this association is understood poorly. The increased risk for type 2 diabetes in depressed patients is believed to result from increased counterregulatory hormone release and action, alterations in glucose transport function, and increased immunoinflammatory activation [52]. These physiologic alterations are believed to contribute to insulin resistance and beta islet cell dysfunction, which ultimately lead to the development of type 2 diabetes [52].

The second hypothesis is that depression in patients who have type 1 or type 2 diabetes results from the chronic psychosocial stressors of having a chronic medical condition [18,53]. This hypothesis is supported by three important studies. In a prospective study, youths who had type 1 diabetes were recruited within 3 weeks of diagnosis and followed over a 10-year period to assess for incident psychiatric conditions [54–56]. Semistructured interviews were conducted at baseline and repeated two to four times per year for 10 years. By the tenth year following a diagnosis of type 1 diabetes, 27.5% had developed major depression.

In another prospective study, 8870 participants from the NHANES Epidemiologic Follow-up Survey who were free of diabetes at baseline were assessed for depression and followed for 9 years [49]. Compared with those who had no depressive symptoms at baseline, those who had high or moderate depressive symptoms did not have a significantly greater incidence of diabetes over the study period. In the Rancho Bernardo study, 1586 older adults were screened for type 2 diabetes with a 75-g oral glucose tolerance test and were screened for depression with a modified Beck's Depression Inventory [57]. There was no evidence that depression was associated with incident diabetes; instead, the study showed that there was a 3.7-fold increased odds of depression in those who had a previous diagnosis of diabetes.

The notion that depression results from chronic psychosocial stressors of having diabetes also is supported by the stress process model [58] and the cognitive adaptation theory [59]. According to the stress process model [58], eventful experiences and chronic life strains create new strains or intensify preexisting strains and produce stress. The stress that results diminishes two aspects of self—mastery and self-esteem—and lead to the development of depression. Mastery refers to the extent to which people see themselves as being in control of forces that have significant impact on their lives, whereas self-esteem involves the individual's judgment about his/her self-worth.

Cognitive adaptation theory argues that in the face of a threatening life event individuals respond with cognitive adaptive efforts that enable them to return to or exceed their previous levels of psychologic functioning [59]. These cognitive adaptive efforts are centered on three themes, which include a search for meaning, an effort to gain mastery of the event, and an attempt to restore self-esteem through self-enhancing evaluations. According to cognitive adaptation theory [59], meaning is dealt with by finding a causal explanation for the experience and restructuring the meaning of life around the event; mastery entails trying to exert behavioral control over the event; and self-esteem is restored by construing personal benefit from the experience and focusing on aspects of the individual's situation that make one seem better off than others in similar situations. Therefore, it is plausible that the diagnosis of diabetes and the daily hassles of managing the disease produce considerable stress that erode positive concepts of self, such as self-esteem and mastery, and can lead to depression, and that patients who have type 2 diabetes who have good cognitive adaptation to the disease—as indicated by high perceived control/mastery, high self-esteem, and high optimism—are less vulnerable to developing depression than are those with poor cognitive adaptation (Fig. 2).

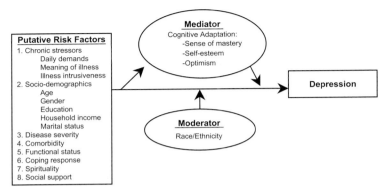

Fig. 2. Conceptual model of the effect of chronic psychosocial stressors and cognitive adaptation on risk for depression in patients who have diabetes.

Review of depression treatment interventions in individuals who have diabetes

Five major clinical trials have been conducted to determine the effectiveness of treatment of depression on depression and diabetes outcomes (Table 2). In the first study, 68 patients who had diabetes and depression were assigned randomly to 8 weeks of treatment with nortriptyline to achieve plasma levels of 50 to 150 ng/mL [60]. Treatment with nortriptyline was associated with significant improvement in mood, but was not associated with significant improvement in glycemic control. In the second study, 51 subjects who had diabetes and depression were randomized to cognitive behavioral therapy plus diabetes education or diabetes education alone [61]. Cognitive behavioral therapy was associated with significant improvements in mood and glycemic control.

In the third study, 60 subjects who had diabetes and depression were assigned randomly to treatment with fluoxetine (up to 40 mg/d) [62]. Treatment with fluoxetine was associated with significant improvement in mood, but was not associated with a statistically significant improvement in glycemic control. The fourth study assessed whether enhancing treatment for depression improved mood and glycemic control in 417 elderly subjects (age ≥ 60 years) who had diabetes and depression [63]. Patients were treated with antidepressants or psychotherapy; a care manager offered education, problem solving, and assistance with medication management; and patients were followed for 12 months. Collaborative care for depression in the elderly improved mood and function but had no significant effect on glycemic control.

The fifth study randomized 329 patients who had diabetes and depression to a case management intervention or usual care to determine whether enhancing the quality of depression care improved depression and diabetes outcomes [64]. The collaborative model of care for depression improved

Table 2
Depression treatment interventions in diabetes: evidence from randomized clinical trials

Intervention (Reference)	Type of diabetes (n)	Effect on depression	Effect on glycemic control	Effect on self-care
Nortriptyline versus placebo 8-wk study (Lustman et al, 1997)	Type 1 (23) Type 2 (45)	Effective (nortriptryline dosed to achieve plasma levels of 50–150 ng/mL)	No statistically significant difference in HbA1c	No significant effect on blood glucose monitoring
CBT + diabetes education program versus diabetes education program alone 10-wk study (Lustman et al, 1998)	Type 2 (51)	Effective (1 h of individual CBT session per wk)	HbA1c decreased by 0.7% in CBT + education group and increased by 0.9% in education alone group at 6-mo follow-up	Adherence to blood glucose monitoring declined in CBT + education group compared to education alone
Fluoxetine versus placebo 8-wk study (Lustman et al, 2000)	Type 1 (26) Type 2 (34)	Effective (fluoxetine in dosages up to maximum of 40 mg/d)	No statistically significant difference in HbA1c	Blood glucose testing was not assessed
Enhanced care for depression versus usual care 12-mo study (Williams et al, 2004)	Type (not specified) (417) Likely type 2 (mean age, 71 y)	Effective (antidepressant—usually SSRI, PST-PC, or antidepressant + PST-PC)	No statistically significant difference in HbA1c	Increase in physical activity in intervention group. No significant difference in adherence to medication, diet, blood glucose testing, or foot care.
Stepped-care for depression versus usual care 12-mo study (Katon et al, 2004)	Type 1 (14) Type 2 (315)	Effective (antidepressant, PST-PC, or antidepressant + PST-PC)	No statistically significant difference in HbA1c	Increase in medication adherence in intervention group

Abbreviations: CBT, cognitive behavioral therapy; HbA1c, glycosylated hemoglobin; PST-PC, problem-solving treatment in primary care; SSRI, selective serotonin reuptake inhibitors.

depression care and outcomes but did not have significant effects on glycemic control. In summary, these studies suggest that collaborative treatment models for depression in people who have diabetes improve depression outcomes but have little to no effect on diabetes outcomes unless some form of diabetes care intervention (eg, diabetes education) is added.

Barriers to effective treatment of depression in individuals who have diabetes

Data suggest that 70% to 90% of patients who have diabetes are treated in primary care settings [65,66]. This means that most diabetic patients who have depression are likely to be treated in primary care settings; however, multiple studies showed that recognition and treatment of depression is less than optimal in primary care settings. Studies showed that only 50% of depressed patients are recognized in primary care settings [67,68]. Even when primary care physicians are alerted to the diagnosis of depression, it does not seem to change treatment patterns [69,70], and most primary care physicians do not escalate doses as needed to achieve complete remission [68,71–73]. Even when patients are started on treatment, a large proportion discontinues their medications within the first 3 months [74,75]. Research suggests that less than 50% of subjects who have major depression and are treated in primary care settings go into remission over a 9- to 12-month period [76,77].

An often overlooked barrier to the early recognition and treatment of depression in diabetic patients is the considerable overlap between symptoms of depression and symptoms of poorly controlled diabetes. Symptoms of depression, such as fatigue, change in weight, change in appetite, or sleep disturbance, overlap considerably with symptoms of diabetes and may hinder the ability of health care providers to recognize clinical depression in patients who have diabetes. The importance of this problem is illustrated by the findings of a recent study [78], which showed that the depression–diabetes symptom association is stronger than is the association of diabetes symptoms with measures of glycemic control and diabetes complications. In that study, patients who had major depression had significantly more diabetes symptoms (Table 3), and the overall number of diabetes symptoms was correlated highly with the number of depressive symptoms.

In addition to barriers that are due to poor recognition, suboptimal dosing, and treatment discontinuation, there are other barriers to effective treatment of depression that are worth mentioning (Box 1). Lingering stigma and inaccurate perceptions about mental illness are important barriers. Stigma may make patients unwilling to acknowledge that they are depressed and may hinder medication adherence. In many cultures erroneous beliefs about the cause of depression is pervasive, and people still see mental illness as a personal failing or a spiritual problem; therefore, there may be a reluctance to initiate treatment or stay on treatment for appropriate periods of time

Table 3
Relationship of major depression to diabetes symptoms adjusted for complications and glycohemoglobin level

Diabetes symptom	Major depression	No major depression	Odds ratio	95% CI
Cold hands and feet	49.4%	32.4%	1.93	1.57–2.38
Numbness in hands or feet	51.3%	32.6%	1.98	1.61–2.43
Pain in hands or feet	46.0%	25.2%	2.23	1.81–2.75
Polyuria	54.5%	33.7%	2.24	1.82–2.75
Excessive hunger	44.7%	20.3%	2.66	2.16–3.28
Abnormal thirst	46.2%	16.9%	3.30	2.67–4.08
Shakiness	39.2%	14.0%	3.33	2.66–4.17
Blurred vision	38.2%	14.2%	3.42	2.74–4.27
Feeling faint	10.9%	2.7%	4.00	2.74–5.86
Daytime sleepiness	84.4%	52.3%	4.96	3.79–6.48

Adapted from Ludman EJ, Katon W, Russo J, et al. Depression and diabetes symptom burden. Gen Hosp Psychiatry 2004;26(6):433.

[79,80]. Other patient-related barriers to treatment include financial constraints, side effects of antidepressants, and implication of a mental health diagnosis on employment and insurability.

Health provider and health systems barriers include insufficient provider knowledge of guideline recommendations, reluctance to escalate dosage, inadequate reimbursement for mental health diagnoses in primary care, and the perceived extra time and effort that are required to deal with mental health issues in primary care settings [81,82]. There also are problems with formulary restrictions in managed care markets and insufficient referral networks in suburban and rural communities.

Fragmentation of care between general health and mental health services and the long-standing practice of packaging mental health services as a "carve-out" program also reduce the overall effectiveness of care. Traditionally, health services for mental health and substance use conditions have been separated from services for general medical conditions, and health care payers typically have sold mental health coverage as separate products to employers and managed care programs. There is growing evidence that lack of a coordinated transition between primary care and specialty mental health care, in part because of the fragmentation and "carve-out" programs, hinders effective treatment and recovery for mental health and substance use conditions [83]. Collectively, these barriers further limit the effectiveness of depression treatment interventions and decrease the likelihood that patients who have diabetes and depression receive high-quality care.

Improving the quality of care: the need for integrated care

The complicated nature of clinical care for diabetes and comorbid depression and the challenge in designing clinical interventions that are effective at

---

Box 1. Barriers to recognition, diagnosis, and optimal treatment of depression

Patient factors
Denial, minimization of symptoms, believing can handle by self
Not seeing depression as medical in nature
Concerns about confidentiality
Not ready to accept diagnosis
Fear of treatments or nonadherence with treatment plan
Stigma of mental health treatment

Physician factors
Not believing it is real illness, serious, or particularly distressing
Interviewing skill deficiencies
Medicalization of symptoms
Fear of offending patient
Knowledge deficit regarding diagnosis or treatment
Diagnosis obscured by comorbidity

Health care system factors
Time constraints
Other pressing clinical issues
Limitations on third-party coverage
Limited treatment resource availability
Restrictions on access to particular treatments
Fragmentation of care

Adapted from Goldman LS, Nielsen NH, Champion HC. Awareness, diagnosis, and treatment of depression. J Gen Intern Med 1999;14(9):577.

---

improving health outcomes for both conditions speaks to the need for integrated models of care for the complex medically ill patient. Interventions that target depression tend to improve depression outcomes alone, whereas interventions that target diabetes tend to improve diabetes outcomes alone. Only one study had clinically significant effects on diabetes and depression; this was due, in part, to the fact that the multifaceted intervention included a depression intervention (cognitive behavioral therapy) and a diabetes intervention (focused diabetes education) [61].

The clinical management of patients who have coexisting diabetes and depression requires collaboration across multiple health care disciplines, including primary care, endocrinology, psychiatry, psychology, nursing, pharmacy, and allied health professions. In most clinical settings, patient care is fragmented and requires referral to practitioners in the different disciplines, who, in most cases, are located at a distance from each other. This fragmentation in care creates major obstacles to achieving good clinical outcomes for patients and works against the provision of high-quality patient care. A coordinated approach to the provision of quality care to people who have diabetes and coexisting depression is needed. This requires widespread implementation of effective strategies to increase recognition of depression, adoption of effective interventions to provide guideline concordant care, and integration of performance measures for depression into diabetes clinical guidelines.

First, it important for primary care practices to implement routine screening for depression for patients who have diabetes. Current guidelines from the U.S. Preventive Services Task Force [84] support the routine use of standardized questionnaires to screen for depression in primary care patients. Ideally, screening should be done yearly. Screening should not take too much additional time if brief screening forms that typically take less than 5 minutes to administer are used. The depression scale of the Patient Health Questionnaire is a brief, valid, and reliable instrument that was developed to screen for depression in primary care [85]. It consists of items that map directly to the American Psychiatric Association's *Diagnostic and Statistical Manual of Mental Disorders, Fourth Edition* [86] criteria for diagnosing major depression and provides a severity measure that can be repeated to guide treatment decisions. Screening alone is not effective unless it is accompanied by effective treatment and follow-up; clinical sites need to have systems in place to screen, confirm, and offer guideline-concordant treatment for depression (Box 2) (also see the article by Kathol and colleagues elsewhere in this issue).

Second, integrated models of care for medically ill patients who have mental health problems need to be adopted more widely. A good example of an integrated care model is the chronic care model [87], which identifies the essential elements of a health care system that encourages high-quality chronic disease management. Health care systems and practices need to implement multidisciplinary health care teams, incorporate evidence-based guidelines into routine clinical practice, and use clinical information systems to provide reminder and feedback to health care providers [88,89]. The widespread implementation of the chronic care model is critical to improving the recognition and treatment of depression in people who have diabetes.

Evidence from the literature supports the chronic care model because studies have shown that interventions to improve the management of depression in primary care need to be multifaceted. A systematic review of educational and organizational intervention to improve the management of depression in primary care found that effective strategies were those with complex interventions that incorporated clinician education, case management by nurses, and greater collaboration between primary care providers and mental health specialists [90].

Third, there is need to integrate performance measures for depression into current treatment guidelines for diabetes. Clinicians and health care

Box 2. Mood disorders in the medically ill: future research, clinical, and public policy agenda

Research
Include depression assessments in all future large-scale
    epidemiologic studies
    Use validated diagnostic instruments
    Include instruments in national population surveys (eg,
        National Health Interview Survey, Medical Expenditure Panel
        Survey, National Health and Nutrition Examination Survey,
        Behavioral Risk Factor Surveillance Survey)
Establish a standardized database
    Standardize diagnostic instruments
    Standardize treatment guidelines
Conduct prospective, rigorously designed studies
    Longitudinal (cohort) studies
    Randomized clinical trials
    Include disease-specific quality of life measures
    Include population pharmacokinetics
Focus on special populations
    Studies on epidemiology, risk, diagnosis, treatment, and
        prevention in minorities, women, children, adolescents, and
        elderly

Clinical
Screen for depression in all medically ill patients
    Screen as part of routine for other indicators of overall health
    Routine screening in primary care and subspecialty clinics
Maintain low threshold for depression treatment
    Provide appropriate treatment early
    Provide patient and family education
    Provide access to additional resources

Public policy
Assess healthcare delivery systems and identify barriers to care
    Document barriers
    Involve professional organizations
    Legislation to provide mental health parity
Confront and reduce the stigma surrounding depression
    Public education programs
    Increase physician awareness
    Peer support programs

Adapted from Evans DL, Charney DS, Lewis L, et al. Mood disorders in the medically ill: scientific review and recommendations. Biol Psychiatry 2005;58(3): 181–2.

systems need to be held more accountable for outcomes of depression and other psychosocial variables in individuals who have diabetes. Incorporation of these performance measures in current guidelines by a variety of agencies and organizations is likely to be more effective in ensuring their widespread adoption and implementation. It also may be important to incorporate diabetes and depression measures in the current pay-for-performance initiatives in the United States. Box 2 summarizes the recommendations of a recent article that reviewed the association between mood disorders and selected medical illnesses, evidence for treatment, and needs in clinical practice and research [91].

Summary

This article reviewed the literature on the adverse health outcomes of the coexistence of diabetes and depression, the challenges of treating coexisting diabetes and depression in a fragmented health care system, and the need for integrated care as a strategy to improve the quality of care for patients who have complex medical illnesses (eg, patients who have coexisting diabetes and depression).

References

[1] National Institute of Diabetes and Digestive and Kidney Diseases. National Diabetes Statistics fact sheet: general information and national estimates on diabetes in the United States, 2003. Bethesda, US Department of Health and Human Services, National Institute of Health; 2003.

[2] National Institute of Diabetes and Digestive and Kidney Diseases. National Diabetes Statistics fact sheet: general information and national estimates on diabetes in the United States, 2003. Revised edition. Bethesda, US Department of Health and Human Services, National Institute of Health; 2005.

[3] King H, Aubert RE, Herman WH. Global burden of diabetes, 1995–2025: prevalence, numerical estimates, and projections. Diabetes Care 1998;21(9):1414–31.

[4] Regier DA, Narrow WE, Rae DS, et al. The de facto US mental and addictive disorders service system. Epidemiologic catchment area prospective 1-year prevalence rates of disorders and services. Arch Gen Psychiatry 1993;50(2):85–94.

[5] Narrow WE. One-year prevalence of depressive disorders among adults 18 and over in the US: NIMH ECA prospective data. National Institute of Mental Health; 1998.

[6] Kessler RC, Berglund P, Demler O, et al. The epidemiology of major depressive disorder: results from the National Comorbidity Survey Replication (NCS-R). JAMA 2003; 289(23):3095–105.

[7] Alonso J, Angermeyer MC, Bernert S, et al. Prevalence of mental disorders in Europe: results from the European Study of the Epidemiology of Mental Disorders (ESEMeD) project. Acta Psychiatr Scand Suppl 2004;(420):21–7.

[8] Demyttenaere K, Bruffaerts R, Posada-Villa J, et al. Prevalence, severity, and unmet need for treatment of mental disorders in the World Health Organization World Mental Health Surveys. JAMA 2004;291(21):2581–90.

[9] Michaud CM, Murray CJ, Bloom BR. Burden of disease–implications for future research. JAMA 2001;285(5):535–9.

[10] US Department of Health and Human Services. Mental Health: A Report of the Surgeon General. Rockville: US Department of Health and Human Services, Substance Abuse and Mental Health Services Administration, Center for Mental Health Services, National Institutes of Health, National Institute of Mental Health; 1999.

[11] Willis T. Diabetes: a medical odyssey. New York: Tuckahoe; 1971.

[12] Lustman PJ, Amado H, Wetzel RD. Depression in diabetics: a critical appraisal. Compr Psychiatry 1983;24(1):65–74.

[13] Robinson N, Fuller JH, Edmeades SP. Depression and diabetes. Diabet Med 1988;5(3): 268–74.

[14] Lustman PJ, Griffith LS, Clouse RE. Depression in adults with diabetes. Results of 5-yr follow-up study. Diabetes Care 1988;11(8):605–12.

[15] Gavard JA, Lustman PJ, Clouse RE. Prevalence of depression in adults with diabetes. An epidemiological evaluation. Diabetes Care 1993;16(8):1167–78.

[16] Anderson RJ, Freedland KE, Clouse RE, et al. The prevalence of comorbid depression in adults with diabetes: a meta- analysis. Diabetes Care 2001;24(6):1069–78.

[17] Egede LE, Zheng D, Simpson K. Comorbid depression is associated with increased health care use and expenditures in individuals with diabetes. Diabetes Care 2002;25(3): 464–70.

[18] Egede LE, Zheng D. Independent factors associated with major depressive disorder in a national sample of individuals with diabetes. Diabetes Care 2003;26(1):104–11.

[19] Lustman PJ, Anderson RJ, Freedland KE, et al. Depression and poor glycemic control: a meta-analytic review of the literature. Diabetes Care 2000;23(7):934–42.

[20] de Groot M, Anderson R, Freedland KE, et al. Association of depression and diabetes complications: a meta-analysis. Psychosom Med 2001;63(4):619–30.

[21] Black SA, Markides KS, Ray LA. Depression predicts increased incidence of adverse health outcomes in older Mexican Americans with type 2 diabetes. Diabetes Care 2003;26(10): 2822–8.

[22] Egede LE. Diabetes, major depression, and functional disability among US adults. Diabetes Care 2004;27(2):421–8.

[23] Egede LE. Effects of depression on work loss and disability bed days in individuals with diabetes. Diabetes Care 2004;27(7):1751–3.

[24] Goldney RD, Phillips PJ, Fisher LJ, et al. Diabetes, depression, and quality of life: a population study. Diabetes Care 2004;27(5):1066–70.

[25] Ciechanowski PS, Katon WJ, Russo JE. Depression and diabetes: impact of depressive symptoms on adherence, function, and costs. Arch Intern Med 2000;160(21):3278–85.

[26] Finkelstein EA, Bray JW, Chen H, et al. Prevalence and costs of major depression among elderly claimants with diabetes. Diabetes Care 2003;26(2):415–20.

[27] Gilmer TP, O'Connor PJ, Rush WA, et al. Predictors of health care costs in adults with diabetes. Diabetes Care 2005;28(1):59–64.

[28] Krapek K, King K, Warren SS, et al. Medication adherence and associated hemoglobin A1c in type 2 diabetes. Ann Pharmacother 2004;38(9):1357–62.

[29] Schectman JM, Nadkarni MM, Voss JD. The association between diabetes metabolic control and drug adherence in an indigent population. Diabetes Care 2002;25(6):1015–21.

[30] Diehl AK, Bauer RL, Sugarek NJ. Correlates of medication compliance in non-insulin-dependent diabetes mellitus. South Med J 1987;80:332–5.

[31] Chousa FP, Guillen VFG, Otero MD, et al. Usefulness of six indirect methods to evaluate drug therapy compliance in non-insulin-dependent diabetes mellitus. Rev Clin Esp 1997; 197:555–9.

[32] Peterson GM, McLean S, Senator GB. Determinants of patient compliance, control, presence of complications, and handicap in non-insulin-dependent diabetes. Aust N Z J Med 1984;14:135–41.

[33] Cramer JA. A systematic review of adherence with medications for diabetes. Diabetes Care 2004;27(5):1218–24.

[34] DiMatteo MR, Lepper HS, Croghan TW. Depression is a risk factor for noncompliance with medical treatment: meta-analysis of the effects of anxiety and depression on patient adherence. Arch Intern Med 2000;160(14):2101–7.

[35] Lin EH, Katon W, Von Korff M, et al. Relationship of depression and diabetes self-care, medication adherence, and preventive care. Diabetes Care 2004;27(9):2154–60.

[36] Kilbourne AM, Reynolds CF III, Good CB, et al. How does depression influence diabetes medication adherence in older patients? Am J Geriatr Psychiatry 2005;13(3):202–10.

[37] American Diabetes Association. Standards of medical care in diabetes. Diabetes Care 2005;28(Suppl 1):S4–36.

[38] Egede LE, Zheng D. Modifiable cardiovascular risk factors in adults with diabetes: prevalence and missed opportunities for physician counseling. Arch Intern Med 2002;162(4):427–33.

[39] Nelson KM, Reiber G, Boyko EJ. Diet and exercise among adults with type 2 diabetes: findings from the third National Health and Nutrition Examination Survey (NHANES III). Diabetes Care 2002;25(10):1722–8.

[40] Harris MI. Frequency of blood glucose monitoring in relation to glycemic control in patients with type 2 diabetes. Diabetes Care 2001;24:979–82.

[41] McKellar JD, Humphreys K, Piette JD. Depression increases diabetes symptoms by complicating patients' self-care adherence. Diabetes Educ 2004;30(3):485–92.

[42] Zhang X, Norris SL, Gregg EW, et al. Depressive symptoms and mortality among persons with and without diabetes. Am J Epidemiol 2005;161(7):652–60.

[43] Egede LE, Nietert PJ, Zheng D. Depression and all-cause and coronary heart disease mortality among adults with and without diabetes. Diabetes Care 2005;28(5):1339–45.

[44] Katon WJ, Rutter C, Simon G, et al. The association of comorbid depression with mortality in patients with type 2 diabetes. Diabetes Care 2005;28(11):2668–72.

[45] Eaton WW, Armenian H, Gallo J, et al. Depression and risk for onset of type II diabetes. A prospective population-based study. Diabetes Care 1996;19(10):1097–102.

[46] Kawakami N, Takatsuka N, Shimizu H, et al. Depressive symptoms and occurrence of type 2 diabetes among Japanese men. Diabetes Care 1999;22(7):1071–6.

[47] Golden SH, Williams JE, Ford DE, et al. Depressive symptoms and the risk of type 2 diabetes: the Atherosclerosis Risk in Communities study. Diabetes Care 2004;27(2):429–35.

[48] Arroyo C, Hu FB, Ryan LM, et al. Depressive symptoms and risk of type 2 diabetes in women. Diabetes Care 2004;27(1):129–33.

[49] Saydah SH, Brancati FL, Golden SH, et al. Depressive symptoms and the risk of type 2 diabetes mellitus in a US sample. Diabetes Metab Res Rev 2003;19(3):202–8.

[50] Carnethon MR, Kinder LS, Fair JM, et al. Symptoms of depression as a risk factor for incident diabetes: findings from the National Health and Nutrition Examination Epidemiologic Follow-up Study, 1971–1992. Am J Epidemiol 2003;158(5):416–23.

[51] van den Akker M, Schuurman A, Metsemakers J. et al. Is depression related to subsequent diabetes mellitus? Acta Psychiatr Scand 2004;110(3):178–83.

[52] Musselman DL, Betan E, Larsen H, et al. Relationship of depression to diabetes types 1 and 2: epidemiology, biology, and treatment. Biol Psychiatry 2003;54(3):317–29.

[53] Talbot F, Nouwen A. A review of the relationship between depression and diabetes in adults: is there a link? Diabetes Care 2000;23(10):1556–62.

[54] Kovacs M, Feinberg TL, Paulauskas S, et al. Initial coping responses and psychosocial characteristics of children with insulin-dependent diabetes mellitus. J Pediatr 1985;106(5):827–34.

[55] Kovacs M, Obrosky DS, Goldston D, et al. Major depressive disorder in youths with IDDM. A controlled prospective study of course and outcome. Diabetes Care 1997;20(1):45–51.

[56] Kovacs M, Goldston D, Obrosky DS, et al. Psychiatric disorders in youths with IDDM: rates and risk factors. Diabetes Care 1997;20(1):36–44.

[57] Palinkas LA, Barrett-Connor E, Wingard DL. Type 2 diabetes and depressive symptoms in older adults: a population-based study. Diabet Med 1991;8(6):532–9.

[58] Pearlin LI, Lieberman MA, Menaghan EG, et al. The stress process. J Health Soc Behav 1981;22(4):337–56.

[59] Taylor SE. Adjustment to threatening events: a theory of cognitive adaptation. Am Psychol 1983;38:1161–73.

[60] Lustman PJ, Griffith LS, Clouse RE, et al. Effects of nortriptyline on depression and glycemic control in diabetes: results of a double-blind, placebo-controlled trial. Psychosom Med 1997;59(3):241–50.

[61] Lustman PJ, Griffith LS, Freedland KE, et al. Cognitive behavior therapy for depression in type 2 diabetes mellitus. A randomized, controlled trial. Ann Intern Med 1998;129(8): 613–21.

[62] Lustman PJ, Freedland KE, Griffith LS, et al. Fluoxetine for depression in diabetes: a randomized double-blind placebo-controlled trial. Diabetes Care 2000;23(5):618–23.

[63] Williams JW Jr, Katon W, Lin EH, et al. The effectiveness of depression care management on diabetes-related outcomes in older patients. Ann Intern Med 2004;140(12):1015–24.

[64] Katon WJ, Von Korff M, Lin EH, et al. The Pathways Study: a randomized trial of collaborative care in patients with diabetes and depression. Arch Gen Psychiatry 2004;61(10): 1042–9.

[65] Harris MI. Medical care for patients with diabetes. Epidemiologic aspects. Ann Intern Med 1996;124(1 Pt 2):117–22.

[66] Egede LE. Association between number of physician visits and influenza vaccination coverage among diabetic adults with access to care. Diabetes Care 2003;26(9):2562–7.

[67] Simon GE, Goldberg D, Tiemens BG, et al. Outcomes of recognized and unrecognized depression in an international primary care study. Gen Hosp Psychiatry 1999;21(2): 97–105.

[68] Katon WJ, Simon G, Russo J, et al. Quality of depression care in a population-based sample of patients with diabetes and major depression. Med Care 2004;42(12):1222–9.

[69] Whooley MA, Stone B, Soghikian K. Randomized trial of case-finding for depression in elderly primary care patients. J Gen Intern Med 2000;15(5):293–300.

[70] Simon GE, Fleck M, Lucas R, et al. Prevalence and predictors of depression treatment in an international primary care study. Am J Psychiatry 2004;161(9):1626–34.

[71] Katon W, von Korff M, Lin E, et al. Adequacy and duration of antidepressant treatment in primary care. Med Care 1992;30(1):67–76.

[72] Lin EH, Katon WJ, Simon GE, et al. Low-intensity treatment of depression in primary care: is it problematic? Gen Hosp Psychiatry 2000;22(2):78–83.

[73] Weilburg JB, O'Leary KM, Meigs JB, et al. Evaluation of the adequacy of outpatient antidepressant treatment. Psychiatr Serv 2003;54(9):1233–9.

[74] Lin EH, Von Korff M, Katon W, et al. The role of the primary care physician in patients' adherence to antidepressant therapy. Med Care 1995;33(1):67–74.

[75] Demyttenaere K, Enzlin P, Dewe W, et al. Compliance with antidepressants in a primary care setting, 1: Beyond lack of efficacy and adverse events. J Clin Psychiatry 2001;62(Suppl 22): 30–3.

[76] Corey-Lisle PK, Nash R, Stang P, et al. Response, partial response, and nonresponse in primary care treatment of depression. Arch Intern Med 2004;164(11):1197–204.

[77] De Almeida Fleck MP, Simon G, et al. Major depression and its correlates in primary care settings in six countries: 9-month follow-up study. Br J Psychiatry 2005;186:41–7.

[78] Ludman EJ, Katon W, Russo J, et al. Depression and diabetes symptom burden. Gen Hosp Psychiatry 2004;26(6):430–6.

[79] Egede LE. Beliefs and attitudes of African Americans with type 2 diabetes toward depression. Diabetes Educ 2002;28(2):258–68.

[80] Cooper-Patrick L, Powe NR, Jenckes MW, et al. Identification of patient attitudes and preferences regarding treatment of depression. J Gen Intern Med 1997;12(7):431–8.

[81] Goldman LS, Nielsen NH, Champion HC. Awareness, diagnosis, and treatment of depression. J Gen Intern Med 1999;14(9):569–80.

[82] Nutting PA, Rost K, Dickinson M, et al. Barriers to initiating depression treatment in primary care practice. J Gen Intern Med 2002;17(2):103–11.

[83] Institute of Medicine. Improving the quality of health care for mental and substance-use conditions: Quality Chasm Series. Washington, DC: National Academy Press; 2006.

[84] US Preventive Services Task Force. Screening for depression: recommendations and rationale. Ann Intern Med 2002;136(10):760–4.

[85] Kroenke K, Spitzer RL, Williams JB. The PHQ-9: validity of a brief depression severity measure. J Gen Intern Med 2001;16(9):606–13.

[86] American Psychiatric Association. Diagnostic and statistical manual of mental disorders. 4th edition. Washington, DC: American Psychiatric Association; 1994.

[87] Wagner EH, Austin BT, Von Korff M. Organizing care for patients with chronic illness. Milbank Q 1996;74(4):511–44.

[88] Bodenheimer T, Wagner EH, Grumbach K. Improving primary care for patients with chronic illness. JAMA 2002;288(14):1775–9.

[89] Von Korff M, Katon W, Unutzer J, et al. Improving depression care: barriers, solutions, and research needs. J Fam Pract 2001;50(6):E1.

[90] Gilbody S, Whitty P, Grimshaw J, et al. Educational and organizational interventions to improve the management of depression in primary care: a systematic review. JAMA 2003; 289(23):3145–51.

[91] Evans DL, Charney DS, Lewis L, et al. Mood disorders in the medically ill: scientific review and recommendations. Biol Psychiatry 2005;58(3):175–89.

ELSEVIER
SAUNDERS

Med Clin N Am 90 (2006) 647–677

THE MEDICAL
CLINICS
OF NORTH AMERICA

Models of Integrated Care

Lawson R. Wulsin, MD[a,*], Wolfgang Söllner, MD[b],
Harold Alan Pincus, MD[c,d,e]

[a]*University of Cincinnati, 231 Albert Sabin Way, ML 559, Cincinnati, OH 45267, USA*
[b]*General Hospital Nürnberg, Prof. Ernst-Nathan-Strasse 1 90419, Nürnberg, Germany*
[c]*Department of Psychiatry, Columbia University, New York, NY*
[d]*New York-Presbyterian Hospital, New York, NY*
[e]*New York State Psychiatric Institute, 1051 Riverside Dr., Unit 09,
New York, NY 10032*

The first formal efforts at the integration of psychiatric and medical care in Europe and North America began in the mid-twentieth century with the psychosomatics movement. An offshoot of psychoanalysis, the psychosomatics movement articulated theoretical bridges between psychiatric and medical illnesses and established some professional societies (American Psychosomatic Society, Academy of Psychosomatic Medicine, German College of Psychosomatic Medicine), but the early integration of psychiatry and medicine was a scholarly endeavor without substantial clinical integration. The integration of psychiatry into medicine on the clinical level began with the emergence in general hospitals of psychiatric consultation and liaison (C-L) services in the 1950s and 1960s in the United States, in the 1970s in Europe, Australia and New Zealand, and in the 1980s in Japan and some Latin American countries such as Brazil and Mexico [1,2]. Although these services first emerged in academic hospital settings, their clinical and economic value soon led to their spread to community and private hospitals. Since the 1970s it has been common in the United States and Europe for large general medical hospitals to provide some form of psychiatric C-L services. In these services consultation services reflect the classic medical consultation model, whereas liaison services aim at a systematic collaboration with a department or ward focused on a specific patient population, including staff education. (In the United Kingdom C-L psychiatric services are

Work for this article was supported in part by RWJF grant #051814 (HAP).
* Corresponding author.
E-mail address: Lawson.wulsin@uc.edu (L.R. Wulsin).

called liaison [psychiatric] services.) In most settings these psychiatric con-sultation services have represented the predominant mental health services available in the medical centers, with other mental health services being se-questered geographically and administratively at other sites. With the rise of cognitive-behavioral therapy and the development of disease management, psychologists have established a clear role in this field, but they suffer the same problems with reimbursement as other mental health clinicians. With the emergence of the clinical practice of C-L psychiatry in the general hospitals came societies, journals, research, and the roots of the subspecialty of psychiatry, now called "psychosomatic medicine' in the United States, aimed at the integration of psychiatry into medicine [1].

A special development took place in Germany where an integrative ap-proach to mental health care emerged inside internal medicine influenced by psychodynamic theoretical backgrounds. In Germany, this approach led to the development of a third medical specialization in mental health care besides general psychiatry and child psychiatry, called "psychosomatic medicine." In contrast to the United States, in Germany psychosomatic medicine is not a subspecialty of psychiatry but a separate medical specialty. In nearly all university hospitals and in an increasing number of general hos-pitals integrated psychosomatic wards and day-hospitals with multiprofes-sional medical teams were established in addition to C-L services [3].

No complementary movement has aimed to run the river the other way and integrate the practice of medicine into psychiatry. That is, there is not yet a formal branch of medicine devoted to the medical problems of people who have mental illness. The provision of medical care in psychiatric hospitals over the past century has fallen to a random group of general practitioners, internists, family doctors, and, in the absence of these, to the psychiatrists em-ployed by the hospitals. No catalyst has brought them together as a group in any formal way, although recent research on the medical aspects of chronic mental illness and its treatments, such as the metabolic syndrome, may finally justify such an organization (see the article in this issue by Gans).

In the past 20 years, however, marked changes in the understanding of the biology of mental illness, the economics of the practice of medicine and psychiatry, and options for training physicians have given birth to new models of integrated care. All these models are young and struggling, but in addition to the C-L model, there now are inpatient medical psychiatry units (MPU), the private practice of combined medicine and psychiatry, outpatient psychiatry practiced in primary care settings, outpatient psychiatry practiced in specialty medical clinics, and outpatient medicine practiced in specialty psychiatry hospitals and clinics. This article describes each of these models, their distin-guishing clinical and financial features, and their relative advantages and disadvantages over traditional practice models. Vignettes about individual practitioners illustrate the current practice of each model, parenthetically suggesting that most people who are qualified to work in one model also choose to work in several other models of integrated care. Although the boundaries between models are not always cleanly drawn, in this article the presentation of these models of integrated care is organized into two broad categories, hospital-based models and outpatient models. In each category, the authors describe the qualifications for practicing in each model, the settings, the patient populations, the relevant financial issues, and the distinguishing advantages and disadvantages of practicing in the model.

The slow march of innovation in the integration of psychiatry and medicine reflects the tension between the demand for and the barriers to integration (see also the article in this issue by Kathol and colleagues). The demand comes from patients and their intuitive desire that their minds, brains, and bodies be treated in concert. They want "one-stop shopping" at the primary care level. On the other hand, the barriers to integration come from the tradition, spawned by stigma, of sequestering mental health services away from medical services, including financially separating mental illness and its treatment. As a result, most physicians and organizations that have attempted to integrate the practice of medicine and psychiatry have run into, and often aground on, substantial economic disincentives. Integration may be frustrated or blocked by employers who purchase health plans, the health plans or insurance companies, disease-management programs, credentialing agencies, billing code practices, hospital administrators, and departmental squabbles over who runs and profits from the combined clinical turf. In the following sections, first the models developed in general hospitals are described; the later sections describe models developed in the primary care arena. The latter are accompanied by conceptual issues that must be taken into account when organizing integrated care.

Hospital-based models

Integration of medicine and mental health treatment programs in the general hospital is increasing worldwide but is not standard care. In hospitals where such integrated treatment programs exist, the extent, quality, and method of integration of care vary from site to site. Generally, the following forms of integration of medicine and mental health emerged. Related to the extent of integration and the medical acuity of the patients treated, Kathol developed a classification starting with "type I" integrated care programs (psychiatric units with basic medical services) with low integration and acuity and reaching to type IV programs with high integration and acuity [4].

Integrated programs, type I

Psychiatric units with medical consultation

Although important for delivering integrated services in psychiatric inpatient units, these models are not discussed in this article. The quality of medical care on psychiatric units remains a matter of concern [5].

Integrated programs, type II

Consultation

The majority of C-L services provide consultation for medical/surgical departments functioning as a "fire brigade" for emergency psychiatric care (Table 1, example 1) [6]. A collaborative study conducted in 11 European countries and including more than 200 consultants and 14,000 referrals showed that more than three quarters of the 56 services investigated had a low consultation rate, between 1% and 2%, and provided psychiatric care mainly for medically ill patients who had urgent psychiatric problems (eg, risk of deliberate self-harm, substance abuse, delirium) [7]. Some services (eg, in the United Kingdom, the Netherlands, Portugal, and Australia) have specially trained nurses included in the C-L team. Participation of psychologists in a multidisciplinary C-L team is rare except in Australia and in psychosomatic services in Germany [8].

Liaison

Liaison, as a more integrated form of cooperation with a named consultant assigned to a specific medical/surgical unit who regularly takes part in case conferences, ward rounds, and further education of medical teams, is rather rare in the delivery of mental health service for medical/surgical units (see Table 1; example 2) [6–8]. In the previously mentioned European study, only a few services (mainly psychosomatic services in Germany and Norway) used a more integrated approach and had a specific focus on somatization and adjustment disorder in the chronically ill. Because of the increased presence in the medical unit, liaison services have higher consultation rates (between 2% and 4%), provide more follow-up visits, and communicate with the outpatient medical care providers [9–11]. This service leads to a more effective long-term treatment of patients who have psychiatric comorbidity and patients who have somatoform disorders [12,13]. One of the aims of liaison services is to support medical teams working in distressing surroundings and caring for a high number of severely ill or dying patients (eg, in ICUs, palliative care wards, burn units, or transplantation units) [14,15]. Although surveys of team members of such units show high satisfaction with this kind of support, controlled trials to show its effectiveness are lacking [16].

Liaison coupled with active case finding and case management

Models of liaison coupled with active case finding and case management have been developed in the United States and in Europe (see Table 1; example 3) [1,17,18]. Recently, a new model to assess the biopsychosocial problems and care needs of each newly admitted patient using the INTERMED method to provide active case management to patients who have high care needs was implemented on some hospital wards in the

Netherlands and Switzerland (see the article in this issue by Stiefel and colleagues) [19,20]. The INTERMED is an empiric, action-oriented decision-support method of detecting complex patients in need of multimodal and coordinated care. The INTERMED consists of a semistructured interview and a rating process performed by trained nurses. Patients who have elevated care needs are routinely discussed during daily case conferences using the results of the INTERMED. Care needs are met by designing an individual treatment plan organized by a multidisciplinary team of internists, nurses, and a C-L psychiatrist and nurse. The results of the INTERMED assessment are electronically documented in the clinical chart and used as part of the letter to the referring general practitioner. In a controlled study involving 644 medical inpatients of the Free University Hospital of Amsterdam, The Netherlands, and using a historic control group of the same wards, patients age 65 years or older provided with this type of integrated care showed better quality of life and a reduced length of hospital stay (16 days versus 11 days) compared with care as usual [21,22]. Other studies are discussed in the article by Stiefel and colleagues in this issue. Although liaison services may constitute an advantage over consultation services in terms of better horizontal integration across disciplines in the hospital and vertical integration across settings in outpatient care, implementation is limited in most countries because of insufficient funding.

Specialist-integrated intervention in specific clinical fields
In-patient. More integrated and multidisciplinary mental health services (including psychologists, nurses, or social workers) have been established in special fields of medicine treating patients who have a high prevalence of psychiatric disorder or psychosocial problems (eg, in psycho-oncology, dialysis, HIV/AIDS units, burn units, and transplantation units) [2,15,23]. Some of these services employ active case finding using standardized instruments for the detection of psychiatric comorbidity coupled with psychiatric/psychosomatic treatment [24–26]. Because of the more systematic service delivery to specific patient populations, consultation rates are much higher than in regular C-L services (10% and higher). An example of such an integrated program is delivered in Europe near Paris, at Ville Evrard, a large public psychiatric hospital. Over the past 15 years the department of internal medicine has provided assessments, consultations, and collaborative management of medical problems. All admissions are seen by the internal medicine service, and management includes primary and secondary prevention regimens as well as acute care. The internists participate with the mental health team in comprehensive treatment planning. It is reported that this approach has "improved the physical health and ... mortality of the patients" [27]. Although such services may provide adequate care for medical inpatients who have psychiatric comorbidity or illness-related distress, most of these services are limited to the general hospital admission and, because of the lack of reimbursement, do not offer follow-up visits or coordination

Table 1
Consultation-liaison services

Location Physician, Job Titles	Setting	Staff	Patient Populations	Interventions	Funding	Innovations, Advantages, and Disadvantages
Example 1: Montevideo, Uruguay R. Cesarco internist, faculty, consultant	Psychosocial Medicine Unit, C-L service, inclusive out-patient clinic, 320-bed hospital	3 MDs. (1 internist, 1 psychiatrist, 1 family medicine practitioner, 20 hrs/wk 2 psychologists, 8 hrs/wk	Medical/surgical patients, liaison with nephrology/dialysis, hemato-oncology, oncology	Consultation rate 2.7%, diagnosis and treatment (pharmacology, counseling), support and education of the medical team, participation in the ethical and cancer committee	Hospital salary (around $US 136) Psychologists are volunteers	Advantage: good acceptance of this biopsychosocial approach, each consult is a opportunity to educate staff. Rotation on unit is required for residents in family medicine Disadvantage: insufficient funding; part-time staffing (full-time staffing nonexistent in the country)
Example 2: Nürnberg General Hospital, Germany W. Söllner general medicine, psychosomaticist and psychiatrist, faculty, consultant	Psychosomatic C-L service in 2200 bed hospital, coordination with psychosomatic ward and day hospital	4 FTE psychosomatic consultants; 3.5 FTE psychologists; social worker	Medical/surgical patients, liaison with oncology, cardiology, dialysis, transplantation, pulmonology, HIV/AIDS, burn unit, dermatology, gynecology, palliative care, geriatrics	2400 cases/yr (consultation rate = 3%); consultations; liaison; counseling of medical teams; communication skills training for medical/surgical physicians; participation in ethical counseling	Consultations are reimbursed by the general budget of the general health; in future, they will be reimbursed by the medical/surgical departments' DRG budgets	Advantage: good integration by liaison, including communication skills training for medical/surgical physicians Disadvantage: separate budgets for mental health and general health; insufficient reimbursement

Example 3: University Medical Center Groningen The Netherlands Department of General Internal Medicine J.P.J. Slaets geriatrician, faculty chair F.J. Huyse, psychiatrist, faculty, consultant integrated care	Admission ward of internal medicine and subsequent wards; outpatient clinic for unexplained physical complaints	0.7 FTE psychiatrist for the development of integrated care; 0.8 FTE nurse practitioner psychiatry; 0.5 FTE rotating resident psychiatry	Patients referred for admission to General Internal Medicine	Admission screening with the INTERMED and subsequent care planning; psychiatric cotreatment when indicated	Primarily as an innovation project but mainly from resources from the Department of General Internal Medicine	Advantage: preventive integrated thinking from the beginning of an admission leading to a remarkable change in attitude of staff towards patients, their clinical problems, and management; maintenance through additional mental health input will remain necessary Disadvantage: appropriate funding is the main problem

Abbreviations: C-L, consultation-liaison; FTE, full-time equivalent; DRG, Diagnosis Related Group.

of care after discharge. This absence of follow-up constitutes a major limitation to treatment continuity and vertical integration.

Outpatient. Outpatient psychiatric treatment programs located at the general hospital were established for specific groups of patients who have chronic disease and who are extensive users of the health care system (eg, patients who have somatization disorder, eating disorders, chronic pain, diabetes associated with eating disorders, or personality disorders causing compliance problems, puerperal psychiatric disorders, and others). Models of integrated care for somatizing patients are described in the article by Kroenke and colleagues in this issue. Some other examples are mentioned here.

An early model of integration of medical and psychiatric care was developed in an general internal medicine clinic where a C-L psychiatrist and a psychologist screened all patients who had unexplained medical symptoms for psychiatric comorbidity and discussed these cases with the internist with a special focus on the communication of the different health care providers involved in the case. Together, they developed a therapeutic strategy and provided a protocol for the telephone case discussion between the internist and the family doctor who provided further treatment. In a randomized, controlled trial including a follow-up examination, this structured model of integrative care showed several advantages compared with care as usual: psychosocial issues were reported more commonly in the discharge letters, more patients received psychologic treatment, patients' depressive symptoms were reduced, and family doctors were more satisfied with the communication with the specialists [28].

Other models of specialist treatment of somatoform disorders have been developed in the United Kingdom. Creed and co-workers [29] established a structured hospital-based outpatient treatment program for patients who had severe irritable bowel syndrome including multidisciplinary assessment, education, and short-term psychodynamic psychotherapy. In a multicenter three-armed randomized trial comparing two interventions (short-term psychotherapy and treatment with paroxetine) with medical care as usual, both interventions reduced physical and psychologic symptoms more effectively and were more cost effective than the control condition. More models relevant to this population are described in later sections on primary care–based models and disease-management and chronic-care models.

Integrated programs, type III and IV

Medical-psychiatric units and psychosomatic units

To meet better the needs of patients who have somatic and psychiatric comorbidity, and especially those who have high acuity of disease, units that permit simultaneous medical and psychiatric treatment have been established in the United States, Canada, and some other countries [26,30]. In the beginning, most of these units were administered through psychiatry using the advantage of reimbursement outside the Diagnosis Related Group system (type III integrated care programs). In the last 10 years, because of the admission of more patients who have more acute illness and restrictions on psychiatric reimbursements, MPUs were established under medical administration but with integrated psychiatric care (type IV programs) (Table 2; example 1). Today, MPUs exist in most university hospitals and many large teaching hospitals in the United States. Kathol and Stoudemire [30] estimate that 2% to 5% of patients admitted to a general hospital and suffering somatic and psychiatric comorbidity would benefit from treatment in a MPU. In practice, the most prevalent psychiatric disorders treated in MPUs are organic mental disorders, depression, and attempted suicide. Length of stay decreased in the last decade from about 20 days to about 10 days. Core features of such units are (1) location in a medical general hospital, (2) provision of a safe medical and psychiatric environment, (3) professional staff trained in both medical and psychiatric illnesses and treatments, and (4) attending physicians with medical and psychiatric training or a combined training.

In suburban Washington, DC, a graduate of the internal medicine psychiatry residency at Duke University has established a group "Med/Psych Hospitalist" practice. This group works in four community hospitals providing inpatient care for patients who have primary medical and secondary psychiatric diagnoses. They cover 10 to 15 inpatients at a time and provide about five psychiatric consultations per week. Dr. Alexander reports, "A med/psych hospitalist should earn 20% more than a regular hospitalist as a starting salary within an established hospitalist practice (20% higher salary for the additional two years of training)." He has, however, encountered resistance from hospitals and hospitalist groups that are reluctant to pay more for an untested model of care. His advice: "First, show them what you can do, then make yourself invaluable, after which you can negotiate a higher salary." The group reports a reduction in adjusted length of stay of 1 day (4.9 versus 5.9) for this med/psych hospitalist model, enough to record a $13,000 profit for the hospital, compared with a $17,000 loss for usual care (J.A. Alexander, personal communication; 2005).

In Germany and in Switzerland the development was opposite: integrated units were founded inside internal medicine as prototypes of an integrated holistic psychosomatic approach [10,31]. These units allowed the simultaneous medical and psychologic diagnosis and treatment of patients who had chronic medical diseases and psychiatric comorbidity or problems of coping with illness. Their populations differ from med/psych units as developed in the United States. The most prevalent disorders treated in these units are affective disorders, somatoform disorders, and adjustment disorders in medical patients. Psychosomatic units embedded in departments of internal medicine constituted attractive clinical models and teaching venues for students and residents to study an integrative biopsychosocial practical approach. This approach contributed to the development of psychosomatic

Table 2
In-patient medical psychiatry units

Center/ Head of Department	Settings Vertical Integration No. Beds	Patient Populations/ Main Physical Diagnoses	Main Psychiatric Diagnoses	No. Beds/ Patients/Yr	Staff	Funding	Innovations, Advantages and Disadvantages
Example 1: Mayo Clinic Psychiatry and Psychology Treatment Center James Rundell, MD, Medical Director of Geriatric and Medical Psychiatry Program	Located in Mayo Psychiatry and Psychology Treatment Center which is on a general hospital campus with 1000 multispecialty beds	Nursing home patients, national referral patients, from medical/ surgical services through C-L service	Dementia, depression, delirium, behavioral dyscontrol secondary to CNS disorders	14 beds, 700 patients/yr	8 physicians, 2 social workers, 1 part-time internist, 1 part-time physician's assistant, psychiatry residents, 1 recreation therapist, clinical pharmacologist; psychology services available	Fully by insurance	Advantages: provides full medical support unless the patient is severely ill; colocated with ECT service; good training setting. Disadvantage: long length of stay, inadequate reimbursement
Example 2: Heidelberg University Hospital W. Herzog, internist and psychosomaticist	Psychosomatic department with 3 in-patient wards (2 type IV, 1 type III); psychosomatic outpatient clinic	Medical in-patients with psychiatric comorbidity, cardiovascular, gastrointestinal diseases	Severe eating disorders, affective disorders, somatoform disorders, adjustment disorders	69 beds,1600 in-patients/yr 2950 out-patients/yr	20 physicians, 10 psychologists	Fully by insurance	Advantage: combination of type III and type IV medical psychiatric units; combination with out-patient clinic Disadvantages. medical and psychotherapeutic training is very time consuming

| Example 3: Berlin University Hospital H.C. Deter, internist and psychosomaticist | Psychosomatic department with allocated psychosomatic beds in the framework of medical wards | Medical in-patients, 78% with psychiatric diagnoses comorbidity, 28% with psychiatric diagnoses only | F4: 44% F3: 26% F5: 27% (mainly eating disorders) F6: 3% F1: 1% | 15 beds, 180 patients/yr | 2.5 FTE physicians, 0.5 FTE psychologist, 1.0 FTE special psychotherapists (art/body therapist) | Fully by insurance | Advantages: Included effective treatment of patients who have somatization disorders and psychiatric disorders with somatic comorbidity; good integration of psychosomatic diagnostic and therapeutic care in all clinical departments of the hospital Disadvantages: nurses have sometimes insufficient training in psychosomatic care |

Abbreviations: CNS, central nervous system; ECT, Electroconvulsive Therapy; FTE, full-time equivalent.

medicine as a separate mental health specialty in 1992. Subsequently, stand-alone psychosomatic units emerged focusing on the treatment of patients who had somatization, eating disorders, and medical patients who had anxiety or affective disorders but, in most cases, with less acute illness [32]. Most of these stand-alone psychosomatic units use a "therapeutic community" approach. At present, the latter type III units are more common than the original type IV psychosomatic inpatient units.

Häuser and co-workers showed clinical and economic advantages of the treatment of complex patients who had psychiatric comorbidity in psychosomatic units as compared with standard treatment in medical units [33].

The department of psychosomatic and general internal medicine at the University of Heidelberg is an integral part of both the Medical University Hospital and the Center for Psychosocial Medicine of Heidelberg University (see Table 2; example 2). With a total of 69 inpatient beds (1600 inpatients/yr), four outpatient clinics (2950 outpatients/yr) and its C-L service (750 consultations/yr), the department covers the whole spectrum of psychosomatic disorders. Patients suffering from physical and psychiatric comorbidity are treated in a setting that provides simultaneous medical and psychosocial diagnosis and treatment [34,35]. In addition, specialized settings for patients who have eating disorders, somatoform disorders, and posttraumatic stress disorders are available. Psychosocial and psychotherapeutic treatment includes psychodynamic, cognitive-behavioral, and systemic approaches in accordance with current treatment guidelines. Preliminary results suggest the effectiveness of this kind of treatment.

Because psychosomatic medicine is a required part of the medical curriculum in Germany, approximately 350 medical students per year are educated in this field using modern teaching techniques. The Berlin allocated-bed model of the psychosomatic department of the University Hospital Charité Campus Benjamin Franklin provides a C-L service for medical and surgical departments (see Table 2; example 3). Additionally, selected patients who have more severe psychiatric comorbidity undergo more intensive specialized psychosomatic diagnosis and treatment in allocated beds of the psychosomatic department in the wards of other clinical departments (internal medicine, neurology, gynecology, surgery). Psychosomatic assessments indicate a broad spectrum of psychiatric and internal diagnoses. Seventy-two percent of 766 patients treated in these allocated psychosomatic beds presented somatic and psychiatric diagnoses, underscoring the need for simultaneous diagnostic and therapeutic proceedings. Twenty-eight percent of patients showed psychiatric diagnoses only. The most frequent psychiatric diagnoses were anxiety disorders, posttraumatic stress disorder, and neurotic disorders (44%), eating disorders and psychiatric conditions contributing to the development of somatic illness (37%), and affective disorders (25.5%). Treatment includes individual psychodynamic psychotherapy, group therapy, stress management training, art therapy, and relaxation training. Mean length of stay is 21 days. An outcome study conducted in 2004 with 139 consecutive patients showed a significant improvement of symptoms [36].

Specialized day hospitals

One consequence of different efforts to improve vertical integration of mental health care was the creation of day hospitals (Table 3). With the exception of services for patients who have chronic pain, these models now are rare in the field of integrated medical and psychiatric care. The advantage of day hospitals is the possibility of providing more intensive, multidisciplinary, and specialized integrated treatment programs for specific patient groups. For example, day hospitals for patients who have chronic pain provide a 3- to 4-week multidisciplinary program specifically tailored for the treatment of small groups of these patients. Such a program includes education, relaxation, physical exercise and sports medicine, work hardening (a form of vocational rehabilitation), and cognitive-behavioral and psychodynamic therapy. A meta-analysis of outcome studies of such multidisciplinary treatment of patients who had chronic pain proved that such programs are the most effective treatment of severe benign chronic pain [37]. Table 3 shows a typical treatment program for patients who have chronic pain at the Nürnberg General Hospital. Vertical integration is promoted by intensive communication with general practitioners, including multidisciplinary case conferences. Similar programs with specific treatment modules are designed for geriatric patients (see Table 3).

Primary care–based models

The historical separation between primary medical care and behavioral health persists in outpatient settings despite epidemiologic evidence regarding the prevalence of behavioral disorders in primary care and research studies showing that many such disorders are under-recognized and are not treated according to evidence-based guidelines in both primary care and behavior health specialty settings [38–40]. Moreover, the high prevalence of general health conditions among the mentally ill and the poor quality of care for general health problems treated in mental health settings have been well documented [41,42]. Clearly, better linked, coordinated, and integrated care models that redefine the interaction between primary care providers and mental health specialists are needed to improve quality of care and health outcomes for this population [43].

Behavioral health services in primary care settings

The first set of models incorporates behavioral health care within primary care settings (or provides better linkages between these two components) and is most appropriate for individuals who have mild-to-moderate

Table 3
Specialized interdisciplinary day hospital

Center Department Head	Setting	Patient Populations	Main Psychiatric Diagnoses	No. Treatment Sites Patients/Yr	Staff	Treatment Program	Innovations, Advantages, and Disadvantages
Nürnberg General Hospital, Germany W. Söllner general medicine, psychosomaticist, and psychiatrist	Interdisciplinary day hospital for (a) patients who have chronic pain and (b) geriatric patients; combined with pain clinic, C-L service, and psychosomatic ward (type III)	(a) Patients who have chronic pain (b) Geriatric patients who have medical illness (eg, stroke and cardiovascular disease)	(a) Psychiatric factors contributing to chronic pain (b) Dementia, depression, adjustment disorder	(a) 10 places, 340 patients (b) 54 places, 1500 patients	(a) Physicians: 0.75 psychosomaticist, 1 anesthesiologist, 0.3 rehabilitation medicine; 0.75 psychologist, 1 physiotherapist, 0.5 ergotherapist, 1 nurse (b) 1 internist, 0.5 psychosomaticist, 0.5 psychologist, physiotherapists, ergotherapists, nurses	(a) 4-wk daily 8-hr group therapy program: education, relaxation, cognitive behavioral therapy, psychodynamic therapy, sports therapy, work hardening (b) Daily 5-hr program (1–4 wk): training of cognitive functions, education, supportive group therapy, physiotherapy, ergotherapy	Innovation: special intensive psychosomatic treatment programs for patients who have chronic pain and geriatric patients Advantage: good vertical integration with outpatient pain clinic, regular case conference with general practitioners, coordination with psychosomatic ward Disadvantage: no outpatient clinic for geriatric patients

behavioral health disorders. In this model, primary care providers continue to have responsibility for general medical care, but they also have in place a systematic capacity to assess a patient's psychosocial problems and strengths and to conduct screenings for both lesser and more severe disorders. In addition, for all psychiatric conditions initially detected or encountered in primary care settings, the primary care provider maintains an ongoing monitoring capacity and communication linkages with any behavioral health specialist involved in the patient's care. For cases of lesser severity or uncomplicated conditions, the primary care provider also has responsibility for a more extensive assessment and initial treatment through medication and limited psychosocial interventions. For a large proportion of the patients who currently are being treated in the behavioral health specialty area, behavioral health specialists located in primary care setting serve as the mainstay of care. There are many advantages to such arrangements. The drop-off resulting from referral to a separate, more distant (and stigmatized) specialist is reduced. Communication between primary care and behavioral health is enhanced both with regard to individual patients and, more importantly, on a general level. Colocation also allows easy, informal "curbside" consultation and an ongoing educational presence that will raise primary care providers' skills in, and awareness of, these issues. Finally, the presence of behavioral health specialists establishes a more effective behavioral health quality-improvement capacity in the practice. As new behavioral technologies (ie, specific interventions to promote healthy habits and prevent physical and mental illness) are developed and made applicable to populations beyond those traditionally considered to have mental disorders, primary care settings will be an important site for their implementation, especially those targeted to populations profiled to be at high risk for specific conditions.

These models can be described along several dimensions [44]. For example as illustrated in Fig. 1, a generalized theory of linkages between the two systems is presented that is not limited to specific care levels or settings but rather reflects the degree of emphasis on three sets of elements:

1. Contractual elements consisting of formal or informal agreements between the two settings, such as patient referral, data sharing, access to patient records, and follow-up procedures, among others
2. Functional elements that include aspects of the relationship actually encountered by the patient through any possible combination of services, ranging from diagnostic evaluation through short- and long-term treatment models
3. Educational elements that serve to establish and reinforce the primary care provider's knowledge and skills in behavioral health or the behavioral health specialist's understanding of general health issues

Based on this framework, six different models can be envisioned. Model 1 is focused principally on contractual elements (ie, an agreement between individual mental health and general health providers or mental health and

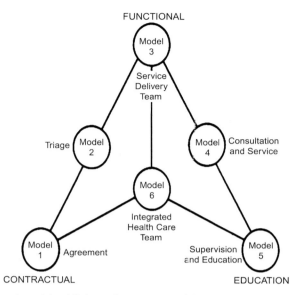

Fig. 1. Conceptual models of linkages between general health and mental health systems of care.

general health organizations regarding referral, information exchange, and other matters). Model 2 adds a person who triages patients and facilitates the contractual arrangements. Model 3 incorporates an actual behavioral health unit that treats most patients who are referred (as in most large health-maintenance organizations). Model 4 places strong emphasis on consulting with the primary care providers, enabling them to treat more of the mental health problems of their patients (as in academically affiliated clinical settings). Model 5 focuses exclusively on education, with no emphasis on service delivery. Model 6 is an integrated health care team wherein the primary care provider and the mental health specialist serve on the same team, treating the patient together. A number of factors need to be taken into account in planning the appropriate type of linkage program for a particular situation or problem. Such factors include the populations to be served, geographical issues, management, financing mechanisms, philosophy of care, and the settings and levels of care. Comparisons should be made across the various models to assess which types of programs are most useful for given situations, which are defined by the above factors.

An alternative set of models can be developed by characterizing the relationship between the primary care provider and the behavioral health specialist along four different dimensions:

1. Who: This dimension is a measure of the extent to which the primary care provider or the behavioral health specialist is involved in the patient's care (Fig. 2)

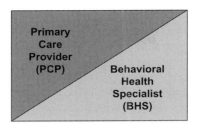

Fig. 2. Who? Responsibility for care.

2. What: This dimension describes the actual functions/roles of each of the providers. Fig. 3 is a matrix providing a sample description of potential underlying assumptions regarding the relevant roles of primary care providers and behavioral specialists (psychiatrists and nonpsychiatrists) for particular conditions. With respect to each condition, cells for specific provider roles and functions are depicted.

3. How: This dimension describes the nature of the relationship between the behavioral health specialist and the primary care provider. Seven possible types of relationships can exist. (1) Integrated team: a single interdisciplinary team provides comprehensive care; (2) collaborative care: both the mental health specialist and the primary care provider are highly involved in the care of the patient as orchestrated through an agreed-upon set of protocols; (3) consultation: the primary care provider

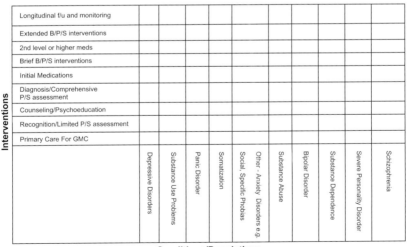

Fig. 3. What? Mapping training to roles. (Does not include pediatric [eg, attention-deficit hyperactivity disorder] or geriatric [eg, dementia] populations. B/P/S, biopsychosocial; f/u, follow-up; GMC, general medical clinic; P/S, psychosocial.

is the principal provider of services but maintains contact and obtains consultation through the mental health specialist; (4) referral: the mental health specialist provides the principal contact, with limited communication with the primary care provider; (5) independent: both the mental health specialist and the primary care provider provide direct patient contact, with no communication between them; (6) autonomous primary care provider: all care is provided by the primary care provider with no involvement or consultation with an mental health specialist; (7) autonomous mental health specialist: all care is provided by the mental health specialist with no involvement or consultation with a primary care provider. These relationships can be operationalized by quantifying communication between the primary care provider and mental health specialist and the extent of mental health specialist patient contact (Fig. 4).

4. When: This dimension describes the points along the patient-care continuum at which the interaction between the primary care provider and mental health specialist occurs (ie, assessment, early management, continuing care) (Fig. 5).

This framework represents a portion (or set of variables) of the full context in which primary care and behavioral health services are delivered. The full set of factors that are likely to affect the process of care and should also be considered includes setting, provider characteristics, patient characteristics, and general health problem issues.

Primary care in behavioral health settings

Most of the time primary care/behavioral health integration is considered from the perspective of integrating behavioral health care into primary care, particularly for individuals who have mild-to-moderate behavioral health

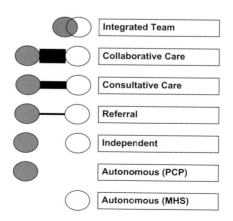

Fig. 4. How? MHC, mental health service; PCP, primary care provider.

Risk Factor Identification/ Prevention	Diagnosis/ Assessment	Short-term Management	Continuing Care

Fig. 5. When?

disorders. There is, however, a compelling need to consider simultaneously alternative models that incorporate the reverse perspective (ie, integrating primary care in behavioral health care for people who have serious behavioral health disorders). Numerous studies over the last 30 years have found high rates of physical health–related problems and death among individuals who have serious mental and addictive disorders [45]. Although some of the excess mortality is a direct result of mental health outcomes (ie, suicide), a substantial proportion is caused by general medical conditions, which often are unrecognized and inadequately treated in this population. Despite their extensive physical health needs, individuals who have behavioral health problems often do not receive treatment. A review of 18 studies estimated that, on average, 35% of individuals who have serious mental disorders have at least one undiagnosed medical disorder. Preventive services, such as vaccinations and cancer screenings, are also lacking. For many of these individuals, especially those treated in the public sector, specialty clinics (eg, community health centers, addiction treatment programs) are the principal or only points of contact with the health care system [41]. For others, primary contact with the health system is through their mental health provider. To improve care for these individuals, it is necessary to go where they are (ie, the specialty mental health system) and bring primary care providers onsite. Such an approach would also allow better integration across other levels of specialty behavioral care and other systems (eg, vocational, welfare, criminal justice), because these connections are better established on the mental health side than in primary care. Numerous efforts are currently underway at state and local levels to implement integrated models of care for these so-called "safety net" populations. The National Council for Community Behavioral Health care has developed a conceptual model to assist providers in thinking about appropriate population-based responses. The Four Quadrant Clinical Integration Model lays out the major system elements that would be used to meet the needs of individuals within four specified quadrants (Fig. 6) [46]:

- Quadrant I: Patients who have low-to-moderate risk/complexity for both behavioral and physical health issues
- Quadrant II: Patients who have high behavioral health risk/complexity and low-to-moderate physical health risk/complexity.

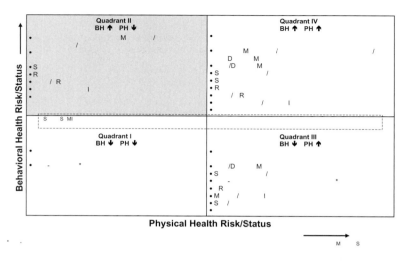

Fig. 6. The four-quadrant clinical integration model. ER, emergency room; IP, inpatient. *From* Mauer BJ. National Council for Community Behavioral Healthcare background paper: behavioral health/primary care integration models, competencies, and infrastructure. © 2002; used with permission. Available at http://www.nccbh.org/SERVICE/consult-pdf/PrimaryCareDiscPaper.pdf.

- Quadrant III: Patients who have low-to-moderate behavioral health risk/complexity and high physical health risk/complexity.
- Quadrant IV: Patients who have high risk/complexity in regard to both behavioral and physical health.

Ongoing public policy efforts will be needed to sustain, support, and mandate integration or coordination of services between behavioral and primary health care services to meet the specialized needs of these various patient populations. To date, a number of integrated and coordinated models of care have been tested and found to achieve some measure of success. In the United States the Bazelon Center for Mental Health Law has examined three basic approaches: (1) embedding of primary care providers within public mental health programs; (2) unified programs that offer mental health and physical health care through one administrative entity, thereby integrating delivery of care and also administration and financing; and (3) initiatives to improve collaboration between independent, office-based primary care and public mental health that use strategies such as special targeted programs, financial incentives, managed-care contract requirements, and provider education and training. On-site demonstrations using the first two approaches have produced excellent results in terms of access, continuity, and coordination of care and have reduced health disparities among people who have serious mental illnesses [45]. There still are policy issues to be resolved regarding service delivery, financing, monitoring, and quality assurance [46]. Possible strategies for resolving these issues might include

providing start-up funds for establishment of embedded or unified programs; stipulating the requirements that must be met by mental health
agencies furnishing on-site primary care; ensuring that reimbursement rates
reflect the cost of providing services and the time spent on care coordination; and placing the responsibility for providing primary care services to individuals who have serious mental illness clearly on one entity [47]. The
third approach has proven to be more difficult because providers continue
to practice separately and have separate administrative structures, information systems, and funding sources. As a result, numerous adjustments and
special efforts to overcome barriers are required. Although efforts to improve collaboration among providers have been somewhat successful,
many problems remain to be addressed through a mix of incentives and
mandates for improving communication, information sharing, financing,
and education.

Disease-management and chronic-care models

As the primary health care system evolves to encompass the management
of chronic diseases in a rapidly aging population, certain behavioral health
disorders have become increasingly recognized as chronic, recurring, and
costly illnesses. The standard of care for virtually all chronic medical
conditions (both physical and mental) now includes the application of disease-specific psychosocial/behavioral interventions ranging from psycho-
education to adherence enhancement to specific cognitive rehabilitation
techniques that alter the course of the disease. Primary care settings have
the responsibility for implementing these interventions and maintaining
the necessary staff and expertise to do so, including behavioral health specialists for interventions that are more complex or technical. Comprehensive
treatment models that approach chronic illness from a longitudinal perspective with systematic monitoring, application of evidence-based models,
active patient engagement, and effective linkages to specialists for consultation and follow-up are also being implemented and tested. Perhaps the best
recognized chronic illness care model (CCM) is the one developed and implemented by Wagner and colleagues that has been applied across a range
of conditions [48,49]. As Fig. 7 illustrates, the Wagner CCM promotes clinical change through six key elements: leadership, decision support, delivery
system redesign, clinical information systems, patient self-management, and
linkage to community resources.

Inherent differences between behavioral and general medical health
require that the CCM be adapted to manage chronic behavioral disorders
effectively. Multiple, large-scale projects testing various adaptations of the
model have demonstrated significant improvement in clinical and economic
outcomes for depression care in particular. Katon and colleagues [50], for
example, empirically tested a CCM-based collaborative care approach designed specifically for depression treatment in primary care that was later

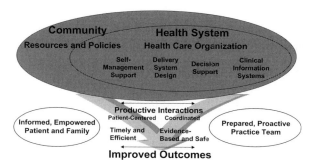

Fig. 7. Evidence-based chronic (planned) care approaches for treating depression.

adapted and proven effective for use by a telephone-based care manager [50–52]. The MacArthur Foundation's Initiative on Depression and Primary Care has launched a variety of projects to explore and enhance current approaches to primary care depression management, including the Re-Engineering Systems for Primary Care Treatment of Depression project, which uses a clinical model for primary care management of depression and a practice change model to support its adoption [53]. As part of the RAND Partners in Care project, Wells [54] also incorporated elements of the Wagner CCM into a broader quality-improvement initiative across diverse managed-care settings. Projects focused on care-management strategies for depression in the elderly, such as the federally funded Prevention of Suicide Primary Care Elderly: Collaborative Trial (PROSPECT) study, Project IMPACT (with support from the John A. Hartford Foundation), the PRISME study (funded by the Substance Abuse and Mental Health Services Administration), and the Quality Enhancement by Strategic Teaming study by Rost and colleagues [55], further substantiate the efficacy of adaptations of the CCM model [55–58]. The Depression in Primary Care program (funded by the Robert Wood Johnson Foundation) attempts to address the barriers to chronic illness primary care for depression through a "6P" strategy that considers the multiple perspectives of the six identified key stakeholder groups (patients, providers, practices, plans/payers, purchasers, and populations) [59]. The incentives component of the program was designed to test the feasibility and effectiveness of combining a clinical CCM with an economic/systems approach to improving the treatment of depression in primary care. Partnerships of primary care practices, health plans (ie, managed-care organizations and managed behavioral health organizations), public and private purchasers, and others are implementing creative interventions for realigning clinical care, organizational structures, and payment incentives and evaluating the effects on organizational processes and outcomes. Other components of the program are designed to support (1) creative and innovative research projects that can document or enhance the value of improving the quality of depression care for the "6P" stakeholders and (2) the efforts of early-career primary care physicians in internal medicine, family medicine, pediatrics, geriatrics, or obstetrics/gynecology in adapting the CCM for depression in their primary care settings.

Systems issues and barriers

Although the need for improved integration of primary medical care and behavioral health care is well documented, and models such as those described previously are being developed and tested, numerous systems issues and barriers continue to impact effective integration adversely at multiple levels, involving all six key stakeholder groups (Fig. 8) [59].

At the patient level, stigma, resistance to diagnosis, and health beliefs that tend to emphasize somatic presentations act as barriers to recognition and treatment of behavioral disorders in the primary care setting. In many cases, the illness itself causes feelings of pessimism, nihilism, and low energy that interfere with help-seeking behaviors or result in unemployment or loss of insurance coverage. For primary care providers, limited time as well as limitations in background, training, and the capacity and interest to reflect introspectively may also act as barriers to appropriate treatment for behavioral health disorders in primary care settings. There is wide variation in how primary care practices are organized to care for people who have behavioral health problems, how they allocate resources in this regard, and how they are linked to behavioral health specialty care. Often there is

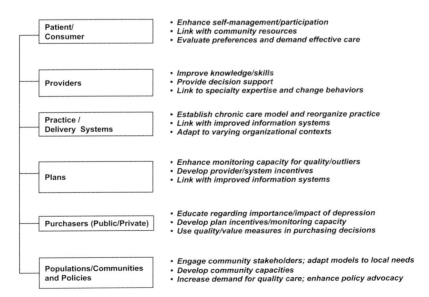

Fig. 8. The "6P" conceptual framework. (*From* Pincus HA, Hough L, Knox Houtsinger J, et al. Emerging models of depression care: multilevel ("6P") strategies. Int J Methods Psychiatric Res 2003;12:54–63; with permission.)

ambiguity about who is responsible for care, and there is limited communication and teamwork between primary care and mental health practices. Typically, primary care practices focus on acute management and referral for what are often chronic or recurrent conditions. Moreover, existing diagnostic systems (ie, *The Diagnostic and Statistical Manual for Mental Disorders-IV*), instruments, and screening tools generally have not been geared toward primary care practice. At the plan/payer level, fragmentation of care through "carve-out" arrangements (ie, in which primary care and behavioral health networks are entirely separate) limit collaboration and communication between primary care and specialty practices and providers and even discourage it with financial and structural disincentives. Approaches for improving care for mental health disorders in both integrated and network managed-care plans have been developed and tested, but these collaborative arrangements are unlikely to remain in place after a demonstration is concluded unless they are tied to financial incentives [60–62]. Although public (eg, Medicare and Medicaid) and private purchasers (eg, business coalitions) exert significant influence over insurance benefit design and coverage decisions, they often fail to consider quality of care as the basis for purchasing decisions. Despite the growing evidence of the increasing value of behavioral health care, awareness of the substantial indirect costs that accrue through absenteeism, presenteeism, and disability remains limited [63]. Behavioral health disorders also place enormous burdens at the population or community level, especially among socially disadvantaged and vulnerable groups. There have not, however, been efforts to link public health approaches more broadly with customized community development models in the service of improving recognition, management, and outcomes [40,48].

Training physicians and nurses in biopsychosocial medicine and communication skills

From the very beginning, one of the aims of C-L psychiatry and psychosomatics was to enhance the biopsychosocial attitudes and communication skills of physicians and nurses to achieve a better holistic care of patients through a "snow-ball effect" created by C-L work [64,65]. The aim of this section is not to review these educational efforts systematically but to provide some examples so that the reader gains an impression of these methods, which may be considered as complementary to the previously mentioned clinical models. Different methods of transferring psychologic knowledge and skills have been developed and integrated in clinical care; among them are the traditional models, such as the so-called "Balint groups" or patient-centered team supervision. More structured approaches appeared more recently, for example the development and implementation of guidelines on specific psychiatric disorders, such as the management of delirium or depression in the medically ill [66]. Although most of these approaches were not evaluated scientifically, training courses developed over the last

2 decades to improve communication skills of physicians and nurses have become the object of scientific interest and have been found highly effective [67]. Such training has been especially developed in two clinical fields in particular, oncology and somatization. Training in communication skills is based mainly on role playing, feedback on audio- or video-taped interviews with simulated patients, and case discussion; designed for oncologists and oncology nurses, they have been successfully implemented and evaluated [68–70]. Training in communication skills is considered relevant and as enhancing patient-centered communication, and the work with videotaped interviews with simulated patients is appreciated. Such training therefore has been developed in different countries, and in one country, Switzerland, is mandatory for oncologists [71].

A comprehensive program has also been introduced at the Memorial Sloan-Kettering Cancer Center in New York City. A dedicated communication skills training and research laboratory has been established at the Memorial Sloan-Kettering Cancer Center, where surgeons, oncologists, nurses, and a range of related clinicians caring for medically ill patients who have cancer are given an applied program of experiential learning. The core program of six modules constitutes a basic oncology curriculum: breaking bad news; discussing prognosis; shared decision making about treatments and clinical trials; responding to distress and anger; transition to palliative care; and obtaining do-not-resuscitate directives and talking with the dying. The consolidation program comprises four modules on geriatric oncology: sensitivity to the elderly; third-party consultations; multidisciplinary teams; and obtaining consent from the cognitively impaired. Other elective modules cover gaining informed consent for phase one trials, genetic risk consultations, working with interpreters, and promoting adherence to treatments. Train-the-Trainer programs ensure facilitators come from the clinical discipline undergoing training. The faculty involved at Memorial Sloan-Kettering Cancer Center expect this training will become the norm for comprehensive cancer centers across the next decade (www.mskcc.org/mskcc/html/44.cfm).

With regard to somatization, the Research Clinic for Functional Disorders and Psychosomatics at Aarhus University Hospital, Denmark, developed a model for training general practitioners to assess and treat patients who present with functional somatic symptoms. The aim of this education model (The Extended Reattribution and Management Model) is to provide knowledge about somatoform disorders and to train general practitioners in interview techniques and communication skills specifically designed for the treatment of patients who have functional disorders [72–74]. The training consists of a 2-day course followed by five follow-up sessions. The program is fitted into a carefully designed research program to assess the effects on the outcome of patients.

In Germany, training courses in basic psychosomatic care, including 20 hours of theoretical seminars, 30 hours of communication skills training, and 30 hours of participation a Balint group, have been broadly implemented during the last decade and now are mandatory for all residents in internal/general medicine.

In the United States Web-based training facilities have been developed (www.impact.ucla.edu) to distribute the methodology of influential studies more effectively [75].

The future of integrated care

The viability of integrated care depends on cultivating a substantial body of evidence from health services research that argues persuasively for the economic and clinical superiority of integrated care over traditional care in specific populations, conditions, or settings. The recently released report of the Institute of Medicine, *Improving the Quality of Health Care for Mental and Substance-Use Conditions: Quality Chasm Series (2006),* provides a blueprint for integrating mental health and general health in the service of improving the quality of all health care [76]. In fact, its principal theme is integration. An entire chapter is devoted to the linkage between these two worlds, and the committee specifically recommends that interventions at multiple levels be applied to move mental health substance use and general health care along a continuum of coordinated care toward horizontal and vertical integration.

The future of integrated care depends in part on resolving the economic barriers to integration. Strategies for resolving theses barriers vary from country to country and, within the United States, even from state to state, because reimbursement rates and credentialing policies can vary by region. In the United States Kathol (www.cartesiansolutions.com) and others have established the process of providing consultations to organizations and individuals aiming to overcome barriers to implementing financially successful programs for psychiatric care in medical settings [47]. For example, most employers have not compared the administrative and claims savings from integrated care with the costs of their traditional "carved out" system. Armed with such internal studies, employers and governmental purchasers of health plans will have more solid grounds for trying new systems that pay for integrated care. In many countries, the organization of health care and particularly separate funding policies for the different components of care hinder the development of successful integration of medical and behavioral care as well as of inpatient and outpatient care.

Kathol [30] defined five critical components for outcome improvement in the integrated care of patients who have medical-psychiatric comorbidity (see also the article by Kathol in this issue):

1. Readily available psychiatric assessment in the primary care setting
2. Active screening in the primary care setting to identify high-risk patients who have psychiatric illnesses/disorders
3. Ability to apply pharmacotherapeutic, psychotherapeutic, and psychosocial interventions that have proven effective through well-designed studies

4. Coordination and integration of medical and psychiatric care among clinicians
5. Case management for patients with chronic or complex illness.

Based on the experienced described previously, the authors add an additional critical component:

6. Support of medical care providers/teams (1) to identify better patients who have medical-psychiatric co-morbidity, (2) to communicate better with these patients and to provide basic psychosocial care and (3) to improve communication within the network of medical care provision.

Depending on the severity and acuity of medical-psychiatric comorbidity and on the degree of complexity of care, a stepped approach to care is necessary, ranging from simple consultation or collaboration between independent medical and psychiatric care providers to more integrated and sophisticated models of care such as MPUs or a combined medical and behavioral outpatient unit. For complex patients mere crisis-oriented consultation is insufficient. The care of such patients requires inpatient or outpatient liaison models with active case finding, assessment of care needs, and interdisciplinary management of care. Interdisciplinary treatment of these patients requires a team approach including medical and behavioral care providers (psychiatrists, psychologists, C-L nurses, nurse case managers, and social workers). Such teamwork requires the development of a common professional culture of integrated care and of interdisciplinary training facilities.

Future models should guarantee sufficient horizontal integration between these care providers in the inpatient or outpatient setting, as well as sufficient vertical integration between inpatient and outpatient care, including forms of transitional care (such as day hospitals and transfer units). Most of the existing models of care do not permit a long-term outcome orientation providing effective referral channels and follow-up strategies. The future models for integrated care will develop along the lines of the models presented in this article. (For models for unexplained physical complaints see also the article in this issue by Kroenke and colleagues; for the chronic care model see also the article in this issue by Egede.) Future models will include complexity assessment to support the decision to assign patient-oriented services and the related levels of care, as discussed elsewhere in this issue.

References

[1] Gitlin DF, Levenson JL, Lyketsos CG. Psychosomatic medicine: a new psychiatric subspecialty. Acad Psychiatry 2004;28(1):4–11.
[2] Levenson J. Introduction. In: Levenson J, editor. Textbook of psychosomatic medicine. Washington (DC): American Psychiatric Publishing, Inc; 2005. p. XIX–XXI.
[3] Herzog T, Hartmann A. [Current status of C–L psychiatry and psychosomatics in West-Germany: a survey]. Nervenartz 1990;61:281–93 [in German].
[4] Kathol RG, Harsch HH, Hall RC, et al. Categorization of types of medical/psychiatry units based on level of acuity. Psychosomatics 1992;33(4):376–86.

[5] Carney CP, Allen J, Doebbeling BN. Receipt of clinical preventive medical services among psychiatric patients. Psychiatr Serv 2002;53(8):1028–30.
[6] Wallen J, Pincus HA, Goldman HH, et al. Psychiatric consultations in short-term general hospitals. Arch Gen Psychiatry 1987;44(2):163–8.
[7] Huyse FJ, Herzog T, Lobo A, et al. Consultation-liaison psychiatric service delivery: results from a European study. Gen Hosp Psychiatry 2001;23(3):124–32.
[8] Huyse FJ, Herzog T, Lobo A, et al. European consultation-liaison psychiatric services: the ECLW Collaborative Study. Acta Psychiatr Scand 2000;101(5):360–6.
[9] Jordan J, Sapper H, Schimke H, et al. [Effectiveness of a patient-centered psychosomatic consultation service. Report of a catamnestic study]. Psychother Psychosom Med Psychol 1989;39(3–4):127–34 [in German].
[10] Deter HC, Weber C, Adolph D, et al. [From applied psychosomatic medicine to integrated medicine—experiences with the Steglitz allocated bed model]. Psychother Psychosom Med Psychol 2004;54(3–4):161–4 [in German].
[11] de Cruppe W, Hennch C, Buchholz C, et al. Communication between psychosomatic C–L consultants and general practitioners in a German health care system. Gen Hosp Psychiatry 2005;27(1):63–72.
[12] Smith GR Jr, Rost K, Kashner TM. A trial of the effect of a standardized psychiatric consultation on health outcomes and costs in somatizing patients. Arch Gen Psychiatry 1995; 52(3):238–43.
[13] Ehlert U, Wagner D, Lupke U. Consultation-liaison service in the general hospital: effects of cognitive-behavioral therapy in patients with physical nonspecific symptoms. J Psychosom Res 1999;47(5):411–7.
[14] Kiss A. Support of the transplant team. Support Care Cancer 1994;2(1):56–60.
[15] Skotzo CE, Stowe JA, Wright C, et al. Approaching a consensus: psychosocial support services for solid organ transplantation programs. Prog Transplant 2001;11(3):163–8.
[16] Herzog T, Stein B, Soellner W, et al. Practice guidelines for consultation-liaison psychosomatics. Stuttgart (Germany): Schattauer; 2002.
[17] Levenson JL, Hamer RM, Rossiter LF. A randomized controlled study of psychiatric consultation guided by screening in general medical inpatients. Am J Psychiatry 1992;149(5):631–7.
[18] Slaets JP, Kauffmann RH, Duivenvoorden HJ, et al. A randomized trial of geriatric liaison intervention in elderly medical inpatients. Psychosom Med 1997;59(6):585–91.
[19] Huyse FJ, Lyons JS, Stiefel FC, et al. "INTERMED": a method to assess health service needs: I. Development and reliability. Gen Hosp Psychiatry 1999;21:39–48.
[20] Stiefel FC, de Jonge P, Huyse FJ, et al. "INTERMED": a method to assess health service needs: II. Results on its validity and clinical use. Gen Hosp Psychiatry 1999;21:49–56.
[21] de Jonge P, Bauer I, Huyse FJ, et al. Medical inpatients at risk of extended hospital stay and poor discharge health status: detection with COMPRI and INTERMED. Psychosom Med 2003;65(4):534–41.
[22] de Jonge P, Latour CH, Huyse FJ. Implementing psychiatric interventions on a medical ward: effects on patients' quality of life and length of hospital stay. Psychosom Med 2003; 65(6):997–1002.
[23] Fawzy FI, Fawzy NW, Arndt LA, et al. Critical review of psychosocial interventions in cancer care. Arch Gen Psychiatry 1995;52(2):100–13.
[24] Hopwood P, Howell A, Maguire P. Screening for psychiatric morbidity in patients with advanced breast cancer: validation of two self-report questionnaires. Br J Cancer 1991;64(2):353–6.
[25] Sollner W, Maislinger S, Konig A, et al. Providing psychosocial support for breast cancer patients based on screening for distress within a consultation-liaison service. Psychooncology 2004;13(12):893–7.
[26] Olbrisch ME, Levenson JL. Psychosocial assessment of organ transplant candidates. Current status of methodological and philosophical issues. Psychosomatics 1995;36(3):236–43.

[27] Saravane D, Vernotte C. [For a multidisciplinary approach in psychiatric somatic care]. Soins Psychiatr 2005;238:8 [in French].

[28] Meeuwesen L, Huyse FJ, Meiland FJ, et al. Psychiatric consultations in medical outpatients with abdominal pain: patient and physician effects. Int J Psychiatry Med 1994;24(4):339–56.

[29] Creed F, Fernandes L, Guthrie E, et al. The cost-effectiveness of psychotherapy and paroxetine for severe irritable bowel syndrome. Gastroenterology 2003;124(2):303–17.

[30] Kathol RG, Stoudemire A. Strategic integration of inpatient and outpatient medical-psychiatry services. In: Rundell TW, editor. The American Psychiatric Publishing textbook of consultation-liaison psychiatry. 2nd edition. Washington (DC): American Psychiatric Publishing, Inc; 2002. p. 871–87.

[31] de Cruppe W, Martens U, Lowe B, et al. [Health service aspects of psychosomatic inpatient treatment in a general hospital]. Psychother Psychosom Med Psychol 2005;55(8):386–91 [in German].

[32] Strauss B, Burgmeier-Lohse M. In-patient and ward psychosomatic psychotherapy: concepts, effectiveness and curative factors. Psychother Psychosom 1993;59(3–4):144–55.

[33] Hauser W, Zimmer C, Klar Y, et al. [Cost effectiveness of integrated internal medicine]. Psychother Psychosom Med Psychol 2004;54(1):34–8 [in German].

[34] Lowe B, Willand L, Eich W, et al. Psychiatric comorbidity and work disability in patients with inflammatory rheumatic diseases. Psychosom Med 2004;66(3):395–402.

[35] Lowe B, Grafe K, Ufer C, et al. Anxiety and depression in patients with pulmonary hypertension. Psychosom Med 2004;66(6):831–6.

[36] Deter HC, Weber C, Adolph D, et al. [From applied psychosomatic medicine to integrated medicine—experiences with the Steglitz allocated bed model]. Psychother Psychosom Med Psychol 2004;54:161–4 [in German].

[37] Flor H, Fydrich T, Turk DC. Efficacy of multidisciplinary pain treatment centers: a meta-analytic review. Pain 1992;49(2):221–30.

[38] Goldman HH, Rye P, Sirovatka P. A report of the Surgeon General. Washington (DC): Department of Health and Human Services; 2000.

[39] Hirschfeld RM, Keller MB, Panico S, et al. The national depressive and manic-depressive association consensus statement on the undertreatment of depression. JAMA 1997;277(4): 333–40.

[40] Wells KB, Miranda J, Bauer M, et al. Overcoming barriers to reducing the burden of affective disorders. Biol Psychiatry 2002;52(6):655.

[41] Druss BG, Rohrbaugh RM, Levinson CM, et al. Integrated medical care for patients with serious psychiatric illness. Arch Gen Psychiatry 2001;58:861–8.

[42] Kilbourne A, Rollman B, Schulberg HC, et al. A clinical framework for depression treatment in primary care. Psychiatr Ann 2002;32(9):1–9.

[43] Pincus HA. The future of behavioral health and primary care: drowning in the mainstream or left on the bank. Psychosomatics 2003;44(1):1–11.

[44] Pincus HA. Patient-oriented models for linking primary care and mental health care. Gen Hosp Psychiatry 1987;9:95–101.

[45] Bazelon Center for Mental Health Law. Get it together: How to integrate physical and mental health care for people with serious mental disorders. Washington (DC): Bazelon Center; 2004.

[46] Parks J, Pollack D, Bartels S, et al. Integrating behavioral health and primary care services: opportunities and challenges for state mental health authorities. National Association of State Mental Health Program Directors Medical Directors Council; 2005. Available at: www.nasmhpd.org. Accessed June 2006.

[47] Bazelon Center for Mental Health Law. Integration of primary care and behavioral health: report on a roundtable discussion of strategies for private health insurance. Washington (DC): Bazelon Center; 2005.

[48] Wagner E, Austin B, Davis C, et al. Improving chronic illness care: translating evidence into action. Health Aff 2001;20:64–78.

[49] Wagner E, Austin B, VonKorff M. Organizing care for patients with chronic illness. Milbank Q 1996;74(4):511–44.

[50] Katon WJ, Robinson P, VonKorff M, et al. A multifaceted intervention to improve treatment of depression in primary care. Arch Gen Psychiatry 1996;53:924–32.

[51] Simon G, Von Korff M, Rutter C, et al. Randomized trial of monitoring, feedback and management of care by telephone to improve treatment of depression in primary care. BMJ 2000; 320:550–4.

[52] Hunkeler EM, Meresman J, Hargreaves WA, et al. Efficacy of nurse telehealth care and peer support in augmenting treatment of depression in primary care. Arch Fam Med 2000;9:700–8.

[53] Dietrich AJ, Oxman TE, Williams JW, et al. Re-engineering systems for the primary care treatment of depression: a cluster randomised controlled trial. BMJ 2004;329(602):605.

[54] Wells KB, Sherbourne CD, Schoenbaum M, et al. Impact of disseminating quality improvement programs for depression in managed primary care. JAMA 2000;283(2):212–20.

[55] Rost K, Nutting P, Smith J, et al. Improving depression outcomes in community primary care practice: a randomized trial of the quEST intervention. Quality Enhancement by Strategic Teaming. J Gen Intern Med 2001;16(3):143–9.

[56] Bruce ML, Ten Have TR, Reynolds CF III, et al. Reducing suicidal ideation and depressive symptoms in depressed older primary care patients: a randomized controlled trial. JAMA 2004;291(9):1081–91.

[57] Unutzer J, Katon W, Sullivan M, et al. Treating depressed older adults in primary care: narrowing the gap between efficacy and effectiveness. Milbank Q 1999;77(2):225–56.

[58] Levkoff SE, Chen H, Coakley E, et al. Design and sample characteristics of the PRISM-E multisite randomized trial to improve behavioral health care for the elderly. J Aging Health 2004;16(1):3–27.

[59] Pincus HA, Houigh L, Knox-Houtsinger J, et al. Emerging models of depression care: multilevel ('6P') strategies. Int J Methods Psychiatr Res 2003;12(1):54–63.

[60] Katon WJ, Von Korff M, Lin E, et al. Collaborative management to achieve depression treatment guidelines. J Clin Psychiatry 1997;58(Suppl 1):20–3.

[61] Meredith LS, Rubenstein LV, Rost KM, et al. Treating depression in staff-model versus network-model managed care organizations. J Gen Intern Med 1999;14(1):39–48.

[62] Simon GE, VonKorff M. Randomised trial of monitoring, feedback, and management care by telephone to improve treatment of depression in primary care. BMJ 2000;320(7234): 550–4.

[63] Schoenbaum M, Kelleher K, Lave JR, et al. Exploratory evidence on the market for effective depression care in Pittsburgh. Psychiatr Serv 2004;55(4):392–5.

[64] Depression in primary care. Linking clinical & system strategies. Robert Wood Johnson Foundation. Available at: www.wpit.edu/dppc/.

[65] Lipowski ZJ. Consultation-liaison psychiatry: the first half century. Gen Hosp Psychiatry 1986;8(5):305–15.

[66] Voellinger R, Berney A, Baumann P, et al. Major depressive disorder in the general hospital: adaptation of clinical practice guidelines. Gen Hosp Psychiatry 2003;25(3):185–93.

[67] Langewitz WA, Eich P, Kiss A, et al. Improving communication skills—a randomized controlled behaviorally oriented intervention study for residents in internal medicine. Psychosom Med 1998;60(3):268–76.

[68] Maguire P, Booth K, Elliott C, et al. Helping health professionals involved in cancer care acquire key interviewing skills—the impact of workshops. Eur J Cancer 1996;32A(9):1486–9.

[69] Razavi D, Delvaux N, Marchal S, et al. The effects of a 24-h psychological training program on attitudes, communication skills and occupational stress in oncology: a randomised study. Eur J Cancer 1993;29A(13):1858–63.

[70] Fallowfield L, Jenkins V. Effective communication skills are the key to good cancer care. Eur J Cancer 1999;35(11):1592–7.

[71] Stiefel F, editor. Communication in cancer care. Recent results in cancer research. Heidelberg (Germany): Springer Verlag, in press.

[72] Fink P, Rosendal M, Toft T. Assessment and treatment of functional disorders in general practice: the extended reattribution and management model–an advanced educational program for nonpsychiatric doctors. Psychosomatics 2002;43(2):93–131.

[73] Frostholm L, Fink P, Oernboel E, et al. The uncertain consultation and patient satisfaction: the impact of patients' illness perceptions and a randomized controlled trial on the training of physicians' communication skills. Psychosom Med 2005;67:897–905.

[74] Rosendal M, Bro F, Sokolowski I, et al. A randomized controlled trial of brief training in assessment and treatment of somatization: effects on GPs' attitudes. Fam Pract 2005;22: 419–27.

[75] Unutzer J, Katon W, Callahan CM, et al. IMPACT: Improving Mood Promoting Access to Collaborative Treatment. Collaborative care management of late-life depression in primary care setting: a randomized controlled trial. JAMA 2002;288(22):2835–45.

[76] Improving the quality of health care for mental and substance-use conditions. Quality Chasm Series. Washington (DC): National Academies Press; 2006.

ELSEVIER
SAUNDERS

Med Clin N Am 90 (2006) 679–692

THE MEDICAL
CLINICS
OF NORTH AMERICA

Case and Care Complexity in the Medically Ill

Peter de Jonge, PhD[a],*, Frits J. Huyse, MD, PhD[b],
Friedrich C. Stiefel, MD, PhD[c]

[a]*Departments of Internal Medicine and Psychiatry, University of Groningen, Hanzeplein 1,
Gebouw 32, P.O. Box 30.001, 9700 RB Groningen, The Netherlands*
[b]*Department of General Internal Medicine, University Medical Center Groningen,
Hanzeplein 1, 9700 RB, Groningen, The Netherlands*
[c]*Service de Psychiatrie de Liaison, Centre Hospitalier Universitaire Vaudois,
Rue du Bugnon 44, CH-1011 Lausanne, Switzerland*

The increasing complexity of health care delivery has been emphasized repeatedly over the last decade [1–7]. In a series of articles in the *BMJ*, an attempt was made to apply complexity science—the scientific reasoning that focuses on the interactions of individual parts that make up a system—to various aspects of health care [1–4]. Plsek and Greenhalgh [1] referred to a complex adaptive system that consists of individual agents with the freedom to act in ways that are not always totally predictable, and whose actions are interconnected so that one agent's actions changes the context for other agents. Although appealingly fitting current general health care, their concepts did not generate much new research and evoked fierce criticism [8]. Because there is ample evidence that patients have become more complex as a result of multimorbidity and that health care systems have become more complex because of subspecialization and new therapeutic techniques, the authors aimed to evaluate the potential use of the concept of complexity for complex patients who have comorbidities.

First of all, a clear definition and measurement strategy of complexity seems to be lacking. Plsek and Wilson [4] described that complexity arises when several systems interact, a situation that seems to be applicable to current health care delivery for patients who have somatic and psychosocial comorbidities; however, not many attempts have been made to define and operationalize complexity in medicine [9]. Complexity should not be mistaken for the absence

---

* Corresponding author.
E-mail address: p.de.jonge@med.umcg.nl (P. de Jonge).

of mathematical modeling or chaos, but rather, as Holden [5] suggested, attention to complexity should reflect a shift in the focus on connections, diversity, and interactions between the agents that are involved in a system.

When focusing on the primary agents that are involved in the health care delivery process (ie, the patient and the health care system in which a health care provider operates), a first clarification of complexity can be made easily—a distinction between "case complexity" and "complexity of care."

Distinction between case and care complexity

It is appealing to distinguish between complexity that arises from characteristics of a patient—such as having multiple interacting diseases that may complicate each other, perhaps with overlap in symptomatology (referred to as case complexity)—and complexity of care that represents aspects of the process of care delivery, such as the involvement of multiple systems and specialties that require interdisciplinary communication to be effective. Although one might assume that complex cases require complex health services, this is not always the case (eg, a patient with multiple diseases who is terminally ill). Conversely, patients who do not have comorbidities may require a complex set of interventions (eg, a patient who develops a cascade of unanticipated treatment complications). Most often, however, a certain match between case and care complexity is needed for efficient health care. Fig. 1 shows how the varying levels of case complexity are managed by corresponding levels of care complexity. To enable such matching between case and care complexity, an operationalization of both is needed that results in a valid tool for effective health care delivery for the complex medically ill.

Case complexity and its assessment

Since the 1980s several attempts have been made to operationalize case complexity by using different perspectives and by aiming at different objectives. A distinction can be made between three groups of case complexity assessment methodologies: patient grouping methodologies, complexity screening instruments, and theoretic constructs.

Patient grouping methodologies

The term "case complexity" or "case mix" has been used most frequently in the area of patient grouping methodologies. Several patient grouping methodologies have been developed to describe discrete clusters of patients [10–13]. Cost containment was the primary incentive for developing such methodologies. Patient grouping methodologies also are used for epidemiologic monitoring, clinical management, comparison of hospital activity, and

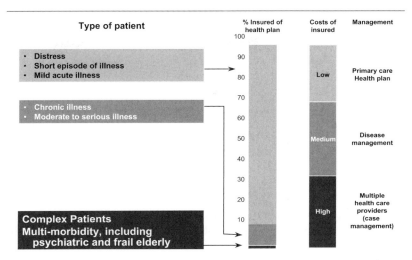

Fig. 1. Matching levels of case complexity to complexity of care in the management of the medically ill.

as a prospective payment system. These systems, such as diagnosis-related groups (DRGs) and case mix groups (CMGs), initially were based solely on medical diagnoses (according to *International Classification of Diseases, Ninth Revision* or *International Statistical Classification of Diseases, Tenth Revision*).

Systems that used medical diagnoses to determine case mix often consisted of too many patient groups, and, more importantly, their predictive ability (of resource consumption) often was limited. As a result, sociodemographic data, severity of illness, comorbidity, and other relevant patient characteristics that predicted resource use were incorporated, which increased their predictive power, yet expanded the number of patient categories. As an example, the currently applied CMG system in Canada consists of 4752 patient subgroups and the APR-DRG system that is applied in the United States consist of 1258 classes.

The use of patient grouping methodologies that are based on medical diagnoses is widespread. Their usefulness in describing case complexity and related resource use is limited because of large differences within diagnosis-based groups. Although they may be sufficient for their intended goal, they do not provide information about individual care needs with sufficient detail. Varying levels of case complexity within specific patient groups that are defined by medical diagnoses would be of interest, but this is not captured by patient grouping methodologies.

Statistical case finding instruments

The limited predictive power of the DRGs stimulated research on predictors of resource use, such as the length of hospital stay (LOS) [14–16]. This research resulted in systems for the assessment of severity of illness and multimorbidity [17–22]. Additionally, several instruments have been developed for the prediction of (aspects of) care use [23]. Three of them are discussed below.

As early as 1977, Glass and colleagues [24] developed an index for predicting a patient's "nonmedical hospital days" (ie, the number of days that a patient stays in the hospital beyond the acute treatment of the admission problem). Their primary goal was cost containment because they were interested in reducing the "misuse" of hospital beds. A risk score (based on a patient's age, need for placement, and mental disorientation) predicted many extended hospital stays.

In an attempt to reduce care use after acute hospital treatment, Evans and colleagues [25,26] developed a risk-screening method that included variables around hospital admission to detect patients who were at risk for nursing home placement, long hospital stay, or readmission. They found that having two or more chronic medical conditions, living alone or being admitted from a nursing home, dependent ambulation, poor mental status, psychiatric comorbidity, previous admission, age older than 75 years, and being unmarried were predictive of care use. An index was developed based on these risk factors, which was used to detect patients who were at risk for nursing home placement, readmission, or lengthy stay.

Finally, the Complexity Prediction Instrument (COMPRI) was developed using 117 items that covered the patient's admission status, a series of clinical predictions by the treating physician and nurse, severity of illness ratings, living/working situation, stress, social support, activities of daily living, health status, somatization, previous health care use, compliance, drug abuse, and emotional state at admission [27,28]. Items that predicted in-hospital resource use, including LOS, were selected on statistical grounds. This resulted in 13 items—six subjective clinical predictions that were made by the doctor and nurse within the first days of a patient's admission and seven other risk factors, including admission status, functional status, and past resource consumption. Similar to the index that was developed by Evans and colleagues, the COMPRI was used to include patients in an intervention study to assess the effects of case management on LOS and quality of life at discharge [29].

Despite the fact that the predictive power of the aforementioned instruments, in terms of care use, exceeds the far more complicated patient grouping methodologies, several disadvantages also exist. First, these instruments were developed for the prediction of outcomes, such as LOS, which are not stable across settings and time. Therefore, it is to be expected that their generalizability may be limited. For example, hospital stays that are not indicated by medical reasons (nonmedical hospital days), may have been different in an era when the average LOS was about 30 days. Second, and perhaps more importantly, these instruments, based on a statistical evaluation of variables, are prospective indicators for resource consumption, but their clinical value in designing interdisciplinary treatment is limited. Although such instruments can be used to allocate certain interventions (eg, case management) to patients who are at risk for increased resource consumption, they cannot be used to guide such interventions.

Theory-driven case complexity assessments

Assessments that are based on theoretic grounds are a third way to approach case complexity. Several concepts have been introduced in the medical literature to describe the interrelations between somatic and psychiatric comorbidities and their effects on outcomes of care (ie, frailty [see also the article by Slaets elsewhere in this issue], neuroticism [see also the articles by Gans and Kroenke and Rosmalen elsewhere in this issue], and the metabolic syndrome [see also the article by Gans elsewhere in this issue]).

The common ground of these concepts is that (1) they are based on multiple indicators, which together results in a continuous score that reflects a unidimensional vulnerability, and (2) substantial debate on their definitions and operationalizations continues to exist.

Frailty

Frailty is described in the geriatric literature to identify older people who are subjected to a general weakness or misbalance [30,31]. Investigators have tried to operationalize frailty as a clinical syndrome that is related causally to disability and comorbidity [32–34]. Most definitions of frailty emphasize multisystem impairments and vulnerability, and describe frailty by a continuous score that consists of multiple indicators. Indicators of frailty should enable clinicians to identify patients who are at risk in community settings and assisted living environments and to target appropriate interventions to mitigate the consequences of frailty. These indicators include weakness, slowness, exhaustion, obesity, cognitive decline, comorbidity, and functional decline. Frailty seems to have a biologic basis and is recognized easily in the clinical setting; however, the debate on its operationalization is ongoing.

Neuroticism

Neuroticism is defined as the tendency to experience negative, distressing emotions and may be one of the factors that underlies poor somatic and psychiatric health [35]. Neuroticism predicts various mental health problems, including anxiety and depression, but also is associated with poor physical health, even after controlling for comorbid psychiatric health problems [36]. Several explanations for this association are mentioned in the literature.

The disability hypothesis states that neuroticism is the result of, not the cause for, health problems. This hypothesis is unlikely to be the sole explanation, because neuroticism is an independent predictor of prospective chronic somatic disorders. According to the symptom perception hypothesis, the association between neuroticism and poor psychiatric and somatic health is due to an altered symptom perception by neurotic persons. According to the psychosomatic hypothesis, a generic liability to ill health, whether somatic or psychiatric, exists that can be captured by the concept of neuroticism. Recently, it was shown in a large, population-based sample (N = 7000) that neuroticism was related to the total number of the most common somatic symptoms that are reported in primary care (eg, heartburn, enteralgia or stomach ache, back or muscle pain, blocked nose, tickling nose, coughing) (Fig. 2) (Rosmalen, unpublished data from SALUT).

In part, the findings supported the symptom perception hypothesis, because the total number of somatic symptoms increased for each increase in neuroticism, even after controlling for sex, age, and psychiatric health (General Health Questionnaire). Because the strongest associations were found between neuroticism and specific psychosomatic symptoms (eg, nausea, fatigue, stomach ache), the authors concluded that the psychosomatic hypothesis gives the best explanation for their findings.

Therefore, neuroticism may be an interesting indicator for a generic liability to health disturbances. Unfortunately, the concept of neuroticism itself and its assessment is a matter of debate because of its nonspecificity and the conceptual overlap with emotional disturbances [37]. As an

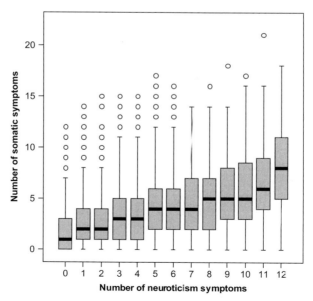

Fig. 2. Level of neuroticism in relation to the number of somatic symptoms. Box length represents the interquartile range, circles represent outliers defined as cases with values greater than 1.5 box lengths from the upper edge of the box.

example, the conceptual overlap between neuroticism and somatization is substantial [38–41].

Metabolic syndrome, depression, and cardiovascular disease

Based on the observation that several of the insulin-related risk factors for cardiovascular diseases are associated, the term "metabolic syndrome" was introduced to describe subjects who are at risk for developing diabetes and heart disease [42]. Since then, several operational definitions have been developed [43–45]. Although there is no doubt about the assumed clustering of risk factors, whether a uniform syndrome exists is still unknown. As an example, the assumption that insulin resistance is the underlying mechanism that defines the metabolic syndrome has not always been confirmed [45]. Conversely, several studies showed that insulin resistance is associated prospectively with cardiovascular morbidity and mortality [46]. Several studies indicated that the metabolic syndrome and insulin resistance also are associated with psychiatric disorders. Most attention has been directed to its association with depression [47–50].

Given the increased prevalence of depression in the presence of diabetes and cardiovascular disease, and the negative prospective association of depression with cardiovascular prognosis in the presence of acute coronary events, an intriguing complex bidirectional association has been hypothesized [51]. Depression is associated prospectively with incident cardiovascular disease, whereas cardiovascular disease is associated prospectively with an increased risk for depression. Although several explanations are possible, the symptom overlap hypothesis (ie, some symptoms [eg, fatigue] can be attributed to depression and to cardiovascular disease) and the shared risk factors hypothesis (depression and cardiovascular disease share certain risk factors, such as vascular risk factors or genotypes) are the most promising.

The symptom overlap hypothesis builds on the longstanding controversy over the diagnosis and treatment of depression in the context of physical illness, which is illustrated by concepts like "somatic depression" [52] and "vital exhaustion" [53–55]. Supporting this hypothesis, the authors found recently that only somatic-affective symptoms of depression—as opposed to cognitive-affective symptoms—were related to cardiovascular prognosis [56]. Somatic-affective symptoms, including fatigue, somatic preoccupation, and work difficulty, were related to clinical depression but also to somatic health status. Mainly, these symptoms were responsible for the often observed association between depression and cardiovascular prognosis, which remained present after controlling for baseline somatic health.

According to the shared risk factors hypothesis [57], the association between depression and cardiovascular disease may be explained by shared (vascular) risk factors for depression and cardiovascular prognosis. The vascular depression hypothesis [57–59] suggests that cerebrovascular lesions due to atherosclerosis play a role in late-life depression. Atherosclerosis is associated with the risk for myocardial infarction and with cardiovascular prognosis. This hypothesis expects that the presence of vascular risk factors is the reason for the association between depression and cardiovascular prognosis. Similarly, the 5-HTTLPR short allele is a genetic risk factor for susceptibility to depression and for cardiac events [60,61]. Therefore, the presence of this genetic marker can explain the bidirectional association between depression and heart disease. Research in the next years might clarify if these shared complaints and shared risk factors are of benefit in targeting patients for interdisciplinary (and preventive) care.

The three theoretic constructs—frailty, neuroticism, and metabolic syndrome—stress the importance of case complexity, irrespective of its expression in somatic or psychiatric morbidity. The advantages of these theory-driven approaches to the assessment of case complexity, when compared with the patient grouping methodologies and the statistical case finders, are that they point to possible mechanisms, and therefore, to possible interventions. The disadvantage is that their relationship with the need for specific interventions is still unclear (ie, the outcomes of these assessments do not necessarily indicate specific treatment actions).

Assessment of complexity of care

Recent findings and developments show that health care systems and professionals should initiate substantial changes to respond to the growing complexity of their organizations; however, in the scientific literature, the attention to complexity of general medical care is limited [62,63]. Moreover, the studies that addressed this topic used perspectives that seem difficult to unify at a first glance.

Indicators of complexity of care include long hospital stay [64], admission to nursing home after discharge [65], nonmedical hospital days [24], and medical complications [21]. Additionally, several studies operationalized complexity of care as the subjectively perceived difficulty of managing patients through the process of health care delivery [62]. Separately, these indicators have been studied extensively. The authors presented an integrated assessment strategy of care complexity using multiple indicators that was validated in a hospital setting using a multisample design. They found that the interrelations of 10 potential indicators of care complexity could be described with a model of four interrelated factors. The model presented below (Fig. 3) describes these interrelations using outcomes of a sample of patients who were admitted to medical wards in seven European countries (N = 2325) [66].

In this model, four aspects of complexity of care—LOS, objective complexity, and complexity perceived by the treating physician and nurse—are assessed by 10 indicators. LOS is the most common measure of hospital functioning; it can be measured easily and reliably and represents a clinical outcome that is related to costs of care. LOS does not address the difficulty of the treatment, however. Therefore, the complexity of care and its

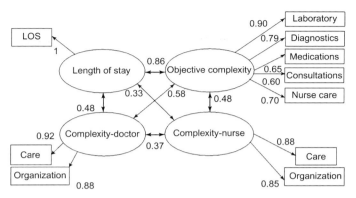

Fig. 3. Measurement model of care complexity. *From* de Jonge P, Huyse FJ, Slaets JPJ, et al. Care complexity in the general hospital: results from a European study. Psychosomatics 2001;42(3):204–12; with permission.

organization also was assessed by surveying the health care professionals— the perception of the treating physician and nurse directly at a patient's discharge. Specifically, a questionnaire was administered that covered several aspects that were related to the complexity of the care and its organization. Because a potential weakness of that method was the subjectivity that was introduced in the assessment, the authors also included several objective indicators that marked the "density" of the care (ie, the number of diagnostic and laboratory tests conducted during the hospital stay, the involvement of consulting specialists, the number of prescribed medications, and the number of specific interventions that were provided by the nursing staff [eg, use of oxygen, nasal tubes. or intravenous lines]).

As anticipated, there was a high correlation between LOS and the objective complexity factor (see Fig. 3). Patients who were in need of many interventions from doctors, nurses, and other medical and paramedical consultants during their hospitalization were likely not to be discharged quickly. The subjectively perceived complexity of care by doctors and nurses was associated strongly with the objective complexity factor. The subjective complexity factors were associated less strongly with LOS and with each other, which highlights different foci of attention. This measurement model of care complexity of patients who were admitted to general medical wards can be summarized as follows. The most central aspect is objective complexity, because it relates most strongly to the three other factors. The indicators of this factor include variables that reflect the actions that took place during the patient's hospital stay that were needed for the diagnosis (laboratory and other tests) and treatment (medications, nursing interventions, consultations with other specialists). As a proxy of this factor, LOS is an adequate index for assessing complexity of care because it is easily accessible and correlates strongly with objective complexity (0.8–0.9). Finally, the clinical relevance of objective complexity is supported by the substantial correlations with both subjective complexity factors (0.5–0.6).

Similar models can be developed as identifiers for complex patients for different health care systems, which, in many cases, could be more simple than this one (see the article by Huyse and colleagues elsewhere in this issue). Such models do not need to be tested formally as the authors did. The goal should be to reach a certain consensus of what care complexity consists of within a given health care setting, so that a link between care complexity and case complexity can be made.

Integrating the assessment of case and care complexity

In the preceding pages, case complexity was distinguished from care complexity, and operational definitions of both were discussed. Ideally, health care systems should adjust the level of care complexity to the level of case complexity to prevent inappropriateness of care. This implies a timely detection of subjects with a high case complexity. Generally, the following strategies are adopted in the general hospital: (1) (non)referral of complex patients by doctors (or nurses), based on their subjective decision, to psychologists, Consultation-liaison psychiatrists, social workers or (psycho)geriatricians, and (2) some form of integrated care that is driven by multidisciplinary rounds, such as postdischarge planning [67–70].

Both options have disadvantages because indications for referral or for multidisciplinary rounds are not operationalized explicitly. Therefore, referrals often are late and urgent, driven by the needs of doctors and nurses; this results in an underdetection of psychiatric comorbidity, which presumably is biased toward patients who represent behavioral problems to the health care professionals [71]. In multidisciplinary rounds, patients may be discussed when there is no need because they are not complex, or patients who are complex are discussed without an adequate conceptualization of their complexity because of a missing assessment tool.

As discussed in the paragraphs on case complexity, patient grouping methodologies, statistical case finding instruments, and the theory-driven case complexity approaches to data have not provided clinically meaningful information. Assessment of care complexity alone, although measurable, cannot guide specific actions and adjustment of care to the complex patient. Until now, an instrument that bridges the gap between case and care complexity, based on empiric research, has been missing. This was the motivation for the authors' group to develop such an instrument [9].

The INTERMED was developed to assess health risks and related health needs (see the article by Stiefel and colleagues elsewhere in this issue) and to adjust the complexity of care to the level of case complexity. Based on an operationalization of the biopsychosocial model that was presented by Engel [72], the INTERMED was not developed to reach a scientific understanding of the causal mechanisms that are involved in case complexity or the interrelations between biologic, psychologic, and social aspects of disease, but to obtain a clinically oriented tool to assist clinicians in identifying complex patients and in designing their interdisciplinary treatment. Still, the items that are included in the INTERMED showed substantial covariance, and, therefore, could be seen as indicators of a generic factor that underlies all variables and together describe the patient's joint vulnerability to biopsychosocial complexity. The INTERMED links the assessment of case complexity with clinical care because it focuses on health care needs and risks. For a detailed discussion of the INTERMED, see the article by Stiefel and colleagues elsewhere in this issue.

Summary

The authors have argued that complexity in general health care is increasingly prevalent because of the increase in patients who have multimorbid conditions, and the increased professional and technical possibilities of medicine. In the increasingly complex care systems, it is necessary—specifically when treating patients in need of integrated care by several providers— that an optimal match between case and care complexity be found in order to prevent poor outcomes in this vulnerable group.

The authors discussed several approaches to case complexity that can be identified in the literature. Most of them seem unsuitable for adjusting case and care complexity, and inadequate for designing multidisciplinary care. Theoretic approaches to case complexity may be of interest, but did not result in clinically meaningful information. The INTERMED, which can be considered the first empirically based instrument to link case and care complexity, is an attempt to improve care delivery and outcomes for the complex medically ill.

References

[1] Plsek PE, Greenhalgh T. The challenge of complexity in health care. BMJ 2001;323:625–8.
[2] Fraser SW, Greenhalgh T. Coping with complexity: educating for capability. BMJ 2001;323: 799–803.
[3] Wilson T, Holt T. Complexity and clinical care. BMJ 2001;323:685–8.
[4] Plsek PE, Wilson T. Complexity, leadership, and management in healthcare organisations. BMJ 2001;323(7315):746–9.
[5] Holden LM. Complex adaptive systems: concept analysis. J Adv Nurs 2005;52(6):651–7.
[6] Aita V, McILvain H, Backer E, et al. Patient-centered care and communication in primary care: what is involved? Patient Educ Couns 2005;58:296–304.
[7] Stewart M. Continuity, care and commitment: the course of patient-clinician relationships. Ann Fam Med 2004;2:388–90.
[8] Reid I. Let them eat complexity: the emperor's new toolkit. BMJ 2002;324:171.
[9] Huyse FJ, Lyons JS, Stiefel FC, et al. Intermed: a method to assess health service needs: I. Development and first results on its reliability. Gen Hosp Psychiatry 1999;21:39–48.
[10] Canadian Institute for Health Information. Acute care grouping methodologies: from diagnosis related groups to case mix groups redevelopment. February 2004. Available at: http://secure.cihi.ca/cihiweb/dispPage.jsp?cw_page = GR_1108_E. Accessed May 2006.

[11] Fetter RB, Shin Y, Freeman JL. Case-mix definition by diagnosis related groups. Med Care 1980;18:1–53.

[12] Averill RF, Muldoon JH, Vertrees JC, et al. The evolution of case mix measurement using diagnosis related groups (DRGs). 1998. Available at: http://www.mmm.com/us/healthcare/his/pdf/reports/evolcasemix5-98.pdf. Accessed May 2006.

[13] Fetter R. Background. In: Fetter R, Brand D, Gamache D, editors. DRGs: their design and development. Ann Arbor (MI): Health Administration Press; 1991. p. 28–42.

[14] Lave JR, Leinhardt S. The cost and length of a hospital stay. Inquiry 1976;13:327–43.

[15] Melfi C, Holleman E, Arthur D, et al. Selecting a patient characteristics index for the prediction of medical outcomes using administrative data. J Clin Epidemiol 1995;48:917–26.

[16] Westert GP, Nieboer AP, Groenewegen PP. Variation in duration of hospital days between hospitals and between doctors within hospitals. Soc Sci Med 1993;37:833–9.

[17] Librero J, Peiro S, Ordinana R. Chronic comorbidity and outcomes of hospital care: length of stay, mortality, and readmission at 30 and 365 days. J Clin Epidemiol 1999;52(3):171–9.

[18] Wright SP, Verouhis D, Gamble G, et al. Factors influencing the length of hospital stay of patients with heart failure. Eur J Heart Fail 2003;5(2):201–9.

[19] Saravay SM, Lavin M. Psychiatric comorbidity and length of stay in the general hospital. Psychosomatics 1994;35:233–52.

[20] Averill RF, McGuire TE, Manning BE, et al. A study of the relationship between severity of illness and hospital cost in New Jersey hospitals. Health Serv Res 1992;27:587–617.

[21] Iezzoni LI, Daley J, Heeren T, et al. Identifying complications of care using administrative data. Med Care 1994;32:700–15.

[22] Wachtel TJ, Derby C, Fulton J. Predicting the outcome of hospitalization for elderly persons: home versus nursing home. South Med J 1984;77:1283–5.

[23] Boult C, Dowd B, McCaffrey D, et al. Screening elders for risk of hospital admission. J Am Geriatr Soc 1993;41:811–7.

[24] Glass RI, Mulvihil MN, Smith H, et al. The 4 score: an index for predicting a patient's non-medical hospital days. American Journal of Public Health 1977;67:751–5.

[25] Evans RL, Hendricks RD, Lawrence KV, et al. Identifying factors associated with health care use: a hospital-based risk screening index. Soc Sci Med 1998;27:947–54.

[26] Evans RL, Hendricks RD. Evaluating hospital discharge planning: a randomized clinical trial. Med Care 1993;31:358–70.

[27] de Jonge P, Huyse FJ, Herzog T, et al. Risk factors for complex care needs in general medical inpatients: results from a European study. Psychosomatics 2001;42(3):213–21.

[28] Huyse FJ, de Jonge P, Slaets JPJ, et al. COMPRI—an instrument to detect patients with complex care needs: results from a European study. Psychosomatics 2001;42(3):222–8.

[29] De Jonge P, Latour C, Huyse FJ. Implementing psychiatric interventions on a general medical ward: effects on patients' quality of life and length of hospital stay. Psychosom Med 2003;65:997–1002.

[30] Winograd CH, Gerety MG, Chung M, et al. Screening for frailty: criteria and predictors of outcomes. J Am Geriatr Soc 1991;39:778–84.

[31] Katz IR. Depression and frailty: the need for multidisciplinary research. Am J Geriatr Psychiatry 2004;12:1–5.

[32] Herrmann FR, Osiek A, Cos M, et al. Frailty judgment by hospital team members: degree of agreement and survival prediction. J Am Geriatr Soc 2005;53(5):916–7.

[33] Rockwood K. Frailty and its definition: a worthy challenge. J Am Geriatr Soc 2005;53(6):1069–70.

[34] Rockwood K. What would make a definition of frailty successful? Age Ageing 2005;34(5):432–4.

[35] Costa PT, McCrae RR. Neuroticism, somatic complaints, and disease: is the bark worse than the bite? J Pers 1987;55:299–316.

[36] Neeleman J, Bijl R, Ormel J. Neuroticism, a central link between somatic and psychiatric morbidity: path analysis of prospective data. Psychol Med 2004;34:521–31.

[37] Ormel J, Rosmalen J, Farmer A. Neuroticism: a non-informative marker of vulnerability to psychopathology. Soc Psychiatry Psychiatr Epidemiol 2004;39(11):906–12.
[38] Gureje O, Simon GE, Ustun TB, et al. Somatization in cross-cultural perspective: a World Health Organization study in primary care. Am J Psychiatry 1997;154(7): 989–95.
[39] Barsky AJ, Ettner SL, Horsky J, et al. Resource utilization of patients with hypochondriacal health anxiety and somatization. Med Care 2001;39(7):705–15.
[40] Fink P, Ornbol E, Toft T, et al. A new, empirically established hypochondriasis diagnosis. Am J Psychiatry 2004;161(9):1680–91.
[41] Creed F, Barsky A. A systematic review of the epidemiology of somatisation disorder and hypochondriasis. J Psychosom Res 2004;56(4):391–408.
[42] Lakka TA, Lakka HM, Salonen JT. Hyperinsulinemia and the risk of coronary heart disease. N Engl J Med 1996;335(13):976–7.
[43] Third report of the National Cholesterol Education Program (NCEP) expert panel on detection, evaluation, and treatment of high blood cholesterol in adults (Adult Treatment Panel III): final report. Circulation 2002;106:3143–421.
[44] Grundy SM, Brewer HB, Cleeman JI, et al. Definition of metabolic syndrome: report of the National Heart, Lung, and Blood Institute/American Heart Association conference on scientific issues related to definition. Circulation 2004;109:433–8.
[45] De Simoni G. State of the art in the metabolic syndrome. Nutr Metab Cardiovasc Dis 2005; 15(4):239–41.
[46] Dekker JM, Girman C, Rhodes T, et al. Metabolic syndrome and 10-year cardiovascular disease risk in the Hoorn Study. Circulation 2005;112(5):666–73.
[47] Kinder LS, Carnethon MR, Palaniappan LP, et al. Depression and the metabolic syndrome in young adults: findings from the Third National Health and Nutrition Examination Survey. Psychosom Med 2004;66(3):316–22.
[48] Timonen M, Laakso M, Jokelainen J, et al. Insulin resistance and depression: cross sectional study. BMJ 2005;330(7481):17–8.
[49] Everson-Rose SA, Meyer PM, Powell LH, et al. Depressive symptoms, insulin resistance, and risk of diabetes in women at midlife. Diabetes Care 2004;27(12):2856–62.
[50] Pouwer F, de Jonge P. Depressive symptoms, insulin resistance, and risk of diabetes in women at midlife: response to Everson-Rose et al. Diabetes Care 2005;28(5):1265–6.
[51] Carney RM, Freedland KE, Miller GE, et al. Depression as a risk factor for cardiac mortality and morbidity: a review of potential mechanisms. J Psychosom Res 2002;53(4): 897–902.
[52] Beck AT, Ward CH, Mendelson M, et al. An inventory for measuring depression. Arch Gen Psychiatry 1961;4:561–71.
[53] McGowan L, Dickens C, Percival C, et al. The relationship between vital exhaustion, depression and comorbid illnesses in patients following first myocardial infarction. J Psychosom Res 2004;57:183–8.
[54] Appels A, Kop W, Bar F, et al. Vital exhaustion, extent of atherosclerosis, and the clinical course after successful percutaneous transluminal coronary angioplasty. Eur Heart J 1995; 16:1880–5.
[55] Wojciechowski FL, Strik JJ, Falger P, et al. The relationship between depressive and vital exhaustion symptomatology post-myocardial infarction. Acta Psychiatr Scand 2000;102: 359–65.
[56] de Jonge P, Ormel J, van den Brink RH, et al. Symptom dimensions of depression following myocardial infarction and their relationship with somatic health status and cardiovascular prognosis. Am J Psychiatry 2006;163:138–44.
[57] Alexopoulos GS, Meyers BS, Young RC, et al. Clinically defined vascular depression. Am J Psychiatry 1997;154:562–5.
[58] Alexopoulos GS, Meyers BS, Young RC, et al. "Vascular depression" hypothesis. Arch Gen Psychiatry 1997;54:915–22.

DE JONGE et al

[59] Alexopoulos GS. Vascular disease, depression, and dementia. J Am Geriatr Soc 2003;51: 1178–80.
[60] Nakatani D, Sato H, Sakata Y, et al. Influence of serotonin transporter gene pclymorphism on depressive symptoms and new cardiac events after acute myocardial infarction. Am Heart J 2005;150(4):652–8.
[61] Williams RB. Treating depression after myocardial infarction: can selecting patients on the basis of genetic susceptibility improve psychiatric and medical outcomes? Am Heart J 2005; 150(4):617–9.
[62] Kelleher C. Relationship of physician ratings of severity of illness and difficulty of clinical management to length of stay. Health Serv Res 1993;27:841–55.
[63] Schoonhoven CB, Scott WR, Flood AB, et al. Measuring the complexity and uncertainty of surgery and postsurgical care. Med Care 1980;18:893–915.
[64] Marchette L, Holloman F. Length of stay: significant variables. J Nurs Admin 1986;16:12–9.
[65] Hickam DH, Hedrick SC, Gorton A. Clinicians's predictions of home placement for hospitalized patients. J Am Geriatr Soc 1991;39:176–80.
[66] de Jonge P, Huyse FJ, Slaets JPJ, et al. Care complexity in the general hospital: results from a European study. Psychosomatics 2001;42(3):204–12.
[67] Institute of Medicine. Crossing the quality chasm: a new health system for the 21st century. Committee on Quality of Health Care in America. Washington DC: National Academy Press; 2001.
[68] Naylor MD, Brooten D, Campbell R, et al. Comprehensive discharge planning and home follow-up of hospitalized elders: a randomized clinical trial. JAMA 1999;281(7):613–20.
[69] Curley C, McEachern JE, Speroff T. A firm trial of interdisciplinary rounds on the inpatient medical wards: an intervention designed using continuous quality improvement. Med Care 1998;36(8 Suppl):AS4–12.
[70] Campion EW. Specialized care for elderly patients. N Engl J Med 2002;346(12):874.
[71] Huyse FJ, Herzog T, Lobo A, et al. Consultation-liaison psychiatric service delivery: results from a European study. Gen Hosp Psychiatry 2001;23(3):124–32.
[72] Engel GL. The need for a new medical mode: a challenge for biomedicine. Science 1977;196: 129–36.

ELSEVIER
SAUNDERS

THE MEDICAL
CLINICS
OF NORTH AMERICA

Med Clin N Am 90 (2006) 693–701

The Complexity of Communication in an Environment with Multiple Disciplines and Professionals: Communimetrics and Decision Support

John S. Lyons, PhD

Psychiatry and Community Medicine, Feinberg School of Medicine, Northwestern University,
Weibolt 717, 339 East Chicago Avenue, Chicago, IL 60611, USA

As discussed in the article in this issue by De Jonge and colleagues, two forms of complexity—the patient's presentation (case complexity) and the application of treatment (care complexity)—are key characteristics that challenge the evolving health care system [1]. Of course, health care environments vary in their complexity. An outpatient practitioner's office is generally considered to be the least complex setting. Hospitals generally provide the most complex care. Even the doctor–patient communication is complicated, but the level of communication complexity in hospital settings is geometrically higher.

Other articles in this issue mention the fragmentation of the health care system. The Institute of Medicine identified the challenge of effective and efficient communication [2]. Many medical mistakes and poor outcomes can be linked to problems resulting from absent, incomplete, or inaccurate communication [3]. Thus processes that support improved communication lie at the core of any systemic solution to the fragmentation of care for medically complex patients [4].

Engel [5] often is credited with the first effort to expand the assessment process beyond the simple identification of a disease process. To date, however, no easy-to-use standard assessment tools have existed to support this expanded biopsychosocial conceptualization of patient care. This article seeks to integrate the conceptualizations of case and care complexity into a measurement strategy to support the conceptual thinking behind this comprehensive approach.

E-mail address: jsl329@northwestern.edu

0025-7125/06/$ - see front matter © 2006 Elsevier Inc. All rights reserved.
doi:10.1016/j.mcna.2006.05.004
medical.theclinics.com

Measurement as communication

Historically, measurement as a field of study has been the enterprise of psychology. Although measurement exists in all science, calibration of laboratory tests and physical assessments are sufficiently straightforward to require limited theory. It is only when the measurement strays from the directly observable that theories of measurement are required to design assessment strategies. When human judgment moderates the direct application of a measure, greater thought must be put into the design of that measure.

Not surprisingly, given the history of measurement, the initial measurement theories have been named "psychometric" theories after the field that developed them. There are several classic texts on psychometric theory. In all of these texts, the goal of communication is listed [6]. In these conceptualizations the communication is among scientists. The goal of communication is to facilitate replication, which is a foundation of scientific progress. Among psychometric theorists, however, communication is much less of a goal relative to reliability and validity.

A number of measures developed from traditional psychometric theories are commonly used in health care. The Medical Outcome Study surveys (eg, Short Form-36, Short Form-12) and Goldberg's General Health Questionnaire stand out as exemplars. It is probably fair to say that such tools have not been routinely applied.

In general, however, measures derived from psychometric theory have failed as standard assessment strategies in service-delivery settings. There are a variety of reasons for this failure, but the two primary ones include the length of these measures (ie, reliability is created by combining less reliable single items into scales) and the need to score the measure before interpretation.

In the mid 1950s Virginia Apgar introduced what was to become known as the first clinimetric measure. As elaborated by Feinstein [7], a clinimetric measure follows the following core principles listed in Box 1.

Box 1. Core principles of a clinimetric measure

- Selection of items is based on clinical rather than statistical criteria.
- No weighting factors are needed; scoring is simple and readily interpretable.
- Variables are selected to be heterogeneous not homogeneous.
- The measure is easy for clinicians to use.
- Face validity is required.
- Subjective states are not measures because they are severely limited in terms of sources of observation.

Thus clinimetric measures involve a single item or a small set of items rated in a fashion that lets the physician know immediately what the implications of a particular score might be. There is no deception in the presentation of the items. There is a complete trust that the individual making the rating is acting in good faith to be as accurate as possible. This approach is very different from that of some psychometric tools that involve self-reporting and that build in validity scales to detect deception.

Over the past decade, the principles of clinimetrics have evolved into a theory of measurement that emphasizes the communication value of the measure (ie, communimetrics). The theory of communimetrics takes the clinimetric approach farther with the additional principles listed in Box 2.

Levels of items translate directly into action levels

The action levels characteristic of communimetric measures influence how individual items are designed. Specifically, anchored definitions are created that are intended to translate immediately into action levels. Several types of action-level ratings have been used. The most common strategy is a four-level rating system with the following action definitions:

0 No evidence. There is no need for action.
1 Watchful waiting/prevention. This need should be monitored, or efforts to prevent it from returning or getting worse should be initiated.
2 Action. An intervention of some type is required because the need is interfering in some notable way with the individual's, family's or community's functioning.
3 Immediate/intensive action. This need is either dangerous or disabling.

Box 2. Additional principles from the theory of communimetrics

- Levels of items translate directly into action levels.
- Measures are reliable at the item level, and ongoing inter-rater reliability is critical to all applications.
- Measures should be malleable to organizational process to fit into service delivery operations with minimal friction.
- A philosophy of "just enough information" drives measure design. An item is included in an application only if it might influence what happens in the service delivery setting.
- All partners involved in the communication process should be involved in the design of the measure.
- The measure must be meaningful to the service-delivery process.
- The value of the measure is determined by its communication utility.

Once an item in a communimetric measure is identified, anchor definitions are created that translate into these four action levels (or into the action levels being used for any specific measure).

Measures are reliable at the item level

There is folklore in the measurement field that there cannot be item-level reliability. That belief is simply not true. Achieving item-level reliability requires the careful design of items, but the author and colleagues have demonstrated that it is possible to achieve item-level reliability with even with relatively long, sophisticated assessment strategies [8]. The many existing clinimetric measures, most of which are single items, also demonstrate the possibility of obtaining item-level reliability. Interrater reliability at the item level is a key requirement of communimetric measures.

Measures should be malleable to the organizational process

Different service-delivery settings operate in different ways. In the more complex settings different individuals serve in different roles that are intended to be coordinated to create efficient and effective care. No two organizations are precisely alike, and the variability in the way health care services are organized across settings can be remarkable. Therefore, any standard approach to measurement must be flexible so that it can be inserted readily into any service-delivery operation at the time that is most opportune for that organization. For example, in some settings the physician must complete any assessments. In other settings nurse practitioners first see the patient and complete certain assessments. In teaching hospitals, residents may have a role in the assessment process. On a different dimension, sometimes the patient is available to participate in the assessment, and sometimes only the family is available. In complex medical environments, a uniform measurement strategy must be flexible to allow assessment to occur regardless of the nature of the informants to the assessment process.

A philosophy of "just enough information" drives measure design

One of the most common complaints physicians and medical staff have about the health care field is the amount of paper work that is required. Documentation requirements vary by settings, but it is clear that health care practitioners' primary interest is in providing health care and not in documenting the provision of their care. Therefore, it is incumbent upon anyone designing a uniform measurement strategy to respect this problem and not require documentation that is not relevant to the work at hand. For this reason, communimetrics allows the addition or deletion of individual items from a measure to fit the information needs of the setting. Because the measures are reliable at the item level, they can be modular so that items can be removed or changed without affecting the reliability or validity of the tool.

All partners involved in the communication process should be involved in the design of the measure

Partner involvement is relatively novel in the field of measurement. Most psychometric measures are created by measurement experts. Although this approach has the advantage of providing statistically sophisticated and psychometrically valid measurement, it has the disadvantage of removing the measurement process somewhat away from the applications. Clinimetric measures generally have been created by practicing physicians. This characteristic has enhanced the meaningfulness of the measure to clinicians. Communimetric measures must be reviewed fully by all partners in the communication process. Thus, if patients and families are an intended target of communication, representatives of this perspective should participate in the development of the measure to ensure that the communication goals are met.

The measure must be meaningful to the service-delivery process

Actual use of the results of a measurement tool in the decision making that occurs in the service-delivery setting is the single most important characteristic to ensure ongoing reliability and validity. If a measure is strictly a documentation requirement, there is risk that reliability might decay over time, particularly if that documentation is not used for ongoing quality-improvement activities. The ideal circumstance is for the measure to provide an information structure that can guide the decision-making process within the service-delivery setting. An example is the use of crisis-assessment tools that support decisions to admit children to the psychiatric hospital or provide community stabilization services [9,10]. These tools provide crisis workers with a framework for understanding the key pieces of information that are important to this decision. As such, the field reliability is high [11].

The value of the measure should be evaluated by its communication utility

Given the different priorities of a communimetric measure, it is important to reconceptualize validity to be consistent with the goals of this measurement approach. Interrater reliability has been mentioned already as a key measurement characteristic. Understandability by all parties using the measure would be a second key characteristic. The relationship of variation in the measure to variation in decision making would be a third. In other words, there should be a clear statistical relationship between scores on the tools and the decisions made in the service-delivery setting. This characteristic would be referred to as "predictive validity" in the psychometric literature. A fourth dimension on which a communimetric measure should be evaluated is the impact of its implementation on the service-delivery process. The use of these tools for decision support and outcomes management should improve the efficiency and effectiveness of service-delivery systems. Without evidence of such effect, there is little reason to continue to use such a measurement approach. The various ways that the impact of a communimetric measure can be evaluated are beyond the scope of this article.

In sum, measurement strategies developed with an emphasis on their communication functions will differ from measures developed emphasizing other priorities. To understand further the potential value of this conceptual shift in how measures are developed, it is useful to explore in detail specific applications of these types of measures.

Decision-support approaches with communimetric tools

One of the notable advantages of measurement approaches developed out of a communimetric framework is that they are easy to apply as decision-support tools. Decision support is a term that describes a set of strategies that are designed to encourage more consistent decision making. In health care and behavioral health care, these applications generally are designed to support decisions about either referral to a specific type of intervention or referral to a specific level of care or intensity of services. The most commonly used decision-support models are for level-of-care/intensity-of-services decision making, although other applications have been studied [8]. With the increased penetration of evidence-based practices in the field, it is likely that models will be widely implemented that support referral to different evidence-based practices.

Before discussing decision support further, it is useful to clarify the distinction between level-of-care decisions and intensity-of-services decisions. Level of care embeds the concept of intensity with the location of the intervention. For example, it is a level-of-care decision to admit to the psychiatric hospital or not. The hospital has 24-hour awake monitoring and daily treatment. The concept of intensity of services is independent of the location of those services. For example, from an intensity-of-services perspective, 24-hour awake monitoring and daily treatment in a home setting is equivalent to psychiatric hospitalization. Most of the existing work in decision support has been with level of care. It is important to note that much of this work is probably equally applicable to intensity of services.

Decision-support strategies

There are essentially two primary strategies that have been used with decision-support approaches—an eligibility approach and a quality improvement approach. Each has advantages and disadvantages, and the choice should be based on the specific circumstances that, it is hoped, will be influenced through the introduction of decision support.

Eligibility models

In eligibility models of decision support, the tool is completed and analyzed before the decision is made. The results of the tool are used to inform the decision before it has been made. In other words, the tool can be used to determine eligibility for different treatments or levels of care. The basic logic of the approach is to use the stepwise process given in Box 3.

Eligibility models of decision support can have powerful impact on an existing service system by creating greater consistency and reducing errors. The downside of an eligibility model is that, in some circumstances, it may be perceived as encouraging "cookie cutter" thinking. Clinical brilliance is the ability to recognize something unique about a case that leads to an approach that differs from the typical treatment. Eligibility systems can discourage clinical brilliance. Thus, establishing appeal processes is an important aspect of managing an eligibility model. In most of the author and colleagues' implementations, appeals run about 2% to 5% depending on the maturity of the system (ie, more mature systems have fewer appeals).

An example of an eligibility model in the general hospital would be any case that involves an automatic referral. For example, an automatic referral to consultation/liaison (C/L) psychiatry for a drug overdose is a simple

---

Box 3. Stepwise approach to designing a decision-support tool

1. Select/develop a measure that captures the key information that ideally should be used to make the target decision.
2. Test the measure on a sample of cases to ensure that it identifies the target population as defined by the following characteristics:
   a. The population has the clinical characteristics for which the program is intended
   b. There is evidence that these individuals actually benefit from receipt of the program/services
   c. The measure does not overly disrupt existing service system by creating radically different decisions (ie, is consistent with the wisdom of the field)
3. Develop the decision-support model on the described sample of cases.
4. Pilot the model with new cases to ensure that it works in practice in a way that is consistent with design intentions.
5. Design an easy, efficient, and fair appeal process for use when partners in the process disagree with the recommended decision.
6. Implement the measure.

example of an eligibility model. Once the assessment that the patient has experienced a drug overdose is made, a referral is made. The C/L psychiatrist or nurse practitioner takes the case from there. The INTERMED method can be used for this type of eligibility referral (see articles in this issue by Huyse and colleagues and Stiefel and colleagues and [12]). The presence of any specific actionable need can generate an automatic referral. Patterns of actionable needs could be used for the intensity of approach.

Quality-improvement models

In the quality-improvement approach to decision support, the tool is completed at the time of the decision, but no analysis/interpretation is done at that time, and no recommendation is made to the deciding clinicians. Rather, feedback is given to these clinicians after a period of time has passed. Using an emergency department process as an example, this feedback could be both individual (eg, "You admitted John to the hospital when most people would not. Why?") or in aggregate (eg, the percentage of low-risk admissions and the percentage of high-risk deflections).

The author and colleagues have used the Severity of Psychiatric Illness measure in a variety of settings for quality-improvement models. Items from the Severity of Psychiatric Illness measure can be used to generate a predictive model of psychiatric admission [9,13] and readmission [14]. These models identify those patients most likely to benefit by hospitalization. They also can be used to understand patterns of use [15]. Once established, these models can be used to understand other factors that interfere with good practice [16].

There are a variety of strategies that can be used to establish models—either clinical or statistical. The clinical strategies involve using the communimetric tool to define the target populations. A psychiatric hospitalization sample, for example, might indicate that patients who have a score of 3 (immediate/intensive action) on the following items:

Psychosis
Danger to self
Danger to others
Self care

And a combined score of 2 (ie, actionable) on any three items would be candidates for psychiatric hospital admission. Further, a score of 2 on psychosis could be added to a score of 3 on medication compliance. As this example indicates, the communimetric measurement approach is a natural fit to a clinical decision-support model, and it naturally divides things out from an action perspective.

Statistical approaches generally involve either the use of logistic regression (for two-category decisions such as admit/no admit) or discriminant function analysis (for decisions with three or more categories). In these models, a development sample is collected in which the decision support tool is collected in the natural environment along with the decision made (unsupported by the assessment). This development sample is used to calculate the statistical relationship between the items of the assessment and the actual decision [9,17]. A prediction model is generated from these data. Next, it is important to test the model on a validation sample of about the same size. This testing is critical, because most statistical approaches maximize the relationship in the development stage, and some "shrinkage" in the prediction accuracy should be expected when the model is applied to a new sample. Too much shrinkage will invalidate the original model.

References

[1] Wilson T, Holt T. Complexity and clinical care. BMJ 2001;323:685–8.
[2] Institute of Medicine. Crossing the quality chasm: a new health system for the 21st century. Committee on Quality of Health Care in America. Washington (DC): National Academy Press; 2001.
[3] Institute of Medicine (2000). To err is human: building a safer health system. Committee on Quality of Health Care in America. Washington (CD): National Academy Press; 2001.
[4] Plesk PE, Wilson T. Complexity, leadership, and management in healthcare organizations. BMJ 2001;323:746–9.
[5] Engel GL. The need for a new medical model: a challenge to biomedicine. Science 1977;196: 129–36.
[6] Nunnally J. Psychometric theory. New York: John Wiley & Sons; 1976.
[7] Feinstein AR. Multi-item 'instruments' vs Virginia Apgar's principles of clinimetrics. Arch Intern Med 1999;159:125–8.
[8] Anderson RL, Lyons JS, West CM. The prediction of mental health service use in residential care. Community Ment Health J 2001;37:313–22.
[9] Lyons JS, Stutesman J, Neme J, et al. Predicting psychiatric emergency admissions and hospital outcome. Med Care 1997;35(8):792–800.
[10] Leon SC, Lyons JS, Uziel-Miller ND, et al. Evaluating the use of psychiatric hospitalization by residential treatment centers. J Am Acad Child Adolesc Psychiatry 2000;39(12):1496–501.
[11] Lyons JS, Rawal P, Yeh I, et al. Use of measurement audit in outcomes management. J Behav Health Serv Res 2002;29(1):75–80.
[12] Huyse FJ, Lyons JS, Stiefel F, et al. Operationalizing the biopsychosocial ,odel. The INTERMED. Psychosomatics 2001;42:1–9.
[13] Mulder CL, van der Graaff PCA, de Jonge P, et al. Predicting admissions in emergency psychiatry. European Psychiatry 2000;15:313.
[14] Lyons JS, O'Mahoney MT, Miller SI, et al. Predicting readmission to the psychiatric hospital in a managed care environment: Implications for quality indicators. Am J Psychiatry 1997; 154:397–400.
[15] Yohanna D, Christopher NJ, Lyons JS, Miller, et al. Characteristics of short-stay admissions to a psychiatric inpatient service. Behavioral Health Service and Research 1998;25:337–46.
[16] Mulder CL, Koopmans GT, Lyons JS. Determinants of indicated versus actual level of care in psychiatric emergency services. Psychiatr Serv 2005;56:452–7.
[17] Lyons JS. Redressing the emperor. Improving our children's public mental health service system. Westport (CT): Praeger; 2004.

ELSEVIER
SAUNDERS

Med Clin N Am 90 (2006) 703–712

THE MEDICAL
CLINICS
OF NORTH AMERICA

Identifiers, or "Red Flags," of Complexity and Need for Integrated Care

Frits J. Huyse, MD, PhD[a],*,
Friedrich C. Stiefel, MD, PhD[b], Peter de Jonge, PhD[c]

[a]*Department of General Internal Medicine, University Medical Center Groningen,*
Hanzeplein 1, 9700 RB, Groningen, The Netherlands
[b]*Service de Psychiatrie de Liaison, Centre Hospitalier Universitaire Vaudois,*
Rue du Bugnon 44, CH-1011 Lausanne, Switzerland
[c]*Departments of Internal Medicine and Psychiatry, University of Groningen, Hanzeplein 1,*
Gebouw 32, Box 30.001, Hanzeplein 1 9700 RB, Groningen, The Netherlands

This issue discusses various aspects of integrated care for multimorbid, complex medical patients. This article presents a practical way to identify patients who are in need of integrated care. Although medically complex patients may constitute an important group, their proportion varies depending on the specific population. Therefore preselection through indicators is almost a conditio sine qua non for effective treatment. In other articles in this issue, arguments are made for screening for psychiatric disease, specifically depression, in patients who have unexplained physical complaints or a chronic disease such as diabetes. A decade ago the authors' group presented a complementary approach, not a disease-specific approach, identifying psychiatric morbidity per se, but one that screens case complexity related to a combination of medical diseases, including psychiatric disorders [1,2]. Therefore a method was needed that could detect and assess case complexity and direct clinical care (see the article by de Jonge and colleagues in this issue). The article by Stiefel and colleagues in this issue discusses such a comprehensive method, the INTERMED method, in detail. Such a method, however, should be used with defined indications.

---

* Corresponding author.
E-mail address: f.j.huijse@int.umcg.nl (F.J. Huyse).

Stepwise screening and assessment model for case complexity

In psychiatric epidemiology, for reasons of cost containment, a two-step procedure is generally used. The COMPRI-INTERMED model may serve as an illustration (Fig. 1) [2]. The Complexity Prediction Instrument (COMPRI), an identifier of complexity and a predictor for negative health care outcomes (Fig. 2) [3–5] precedes the more comprehensive assessment of complexity in terms of care risks and care needs; the INTERMED method [6,7].

Following complexity screening with the COMPRI, the INTERMED method provides meaningful clinical information to direct interdisciplinary care and therefore matches the needs of medically complex patients with the resources of the health care system. For example, it is evident that depression in the medically ill is a major issue, specifically in patients who have chronic diseases and those who have unexplained physical complaints. In the same patient groups, however, anxiety, substance abuse, or cognitive disorders, rather than depression, might be the primary psychiatric

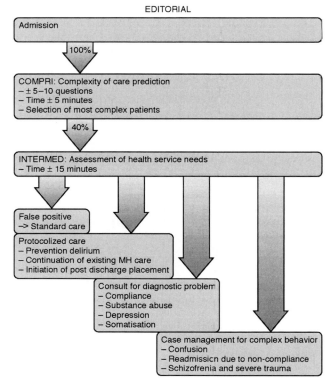

Fig. 1. Stepwise screening and assessment model for case complexity. (*From* Huyse FJ. From consultation to complexity of care prediction and health service needs assessment [editorial]. J Psychosomatic Res 1997;43:233–40; with permission.)

Predictions Made by the Doctor

Do you expect this patient to have a hospital stay of 2 weeks or more?	Yes	No
Do you think the organization of care during hospital stay will be complex?	Yes	No
Do you expect that this patient's mental health will be disturbed during this hospital stay?	Yes	No

Predictions Made by the Nurse

Do you expect this patient to have a hospital stay of 2 weeks or more?	Yes	No
Do you think the organization of care during hospital stay will be complex?	Yes	No
Do you think this patient will be limited in activities of daily living after discharge?	Yes	No

Additional Questions

Is this an unplanned admission?	Yes	No
Is the patient retired?	Yes	No
Is the patient known to have a currently active malignancy?	Yes	No
Did the patient		
have walking difficulties during the last 3 months?	Yes	No
have a negative health perception during the last week?	Yes	No
have more than 6 doctor visits during the last three months?	Yes	No
take more than three different kinds of medications the day prior to admission?	Yes	No

Fig. 2. Complexity prediction instrument. (*From* Huyse FJ, de Jonge P, Slaets JP, et al. COMPRI—an instrument to detect patients with complex care needs: Results from a European study. Psychosomatics 2001;42(3):222–8; with permission.)

disturbance leading to specific complexities. Whereas depression screening has a disease-specific focus that is limited in detectig other psychiatric disorders or social morbidities, complexity screening and assessment has a generic focus and therefore can be used in all patient populations.

Factors influencing the use of complexity indicators

A medical team's awareness of the development of integrated care for complex patients is the most important factor. The recognition that fragmented care for a subgroup of patients served—the complex medically ill—does not deliver adequate services is crucial. Without recognition, there can be no integrated care, and no integrated care is possible without appropriate reimbursement, which is the second factor influencing the use of complexity indicators. It therefore is of utmost importance that all parties involved—clinicians, politicians, health care policy makers, third-party payors (insurance companies), providers, and patients (ie, the parties mentioned in the report of the Committee on Quality of Care of the Institute of Medicine) become aware of the need to develop high-quality integrated care for complex patients [8].

A third factor determining the use of identifier for complexity is population characteristics, such as extent of psychiatric comorbidity or the level of frailty or complexity. The proportion of complex patients depends on the type of patients seen (eg, patients who have diabetes or cardiac disease) and the type of services delivered (eg, primary care or a general hospital acute admission ward). For instance, in a transplant population one might assume that about half of the population will have additional physical morbidities, and the risk of psychologic distress or psychiatric morbidities is high in such a population [9]. Therefore in such a population all patients might qualify for complexity assessment, which would allow formulation of patient-oriented care plans in a highly stressed population that has somatic and psychiatric comorbidities, reduce unpredicted events and negative outcomes. In such a population the indication for transplantation qualifies the patient for a complexity assessment. The planned transplantation is already the identifier, or the "red flag," indicating the need for complexity assessment. In other populations such an assessment might be desirable but not feasible or cost effective for the entire population.

A fourth factor to be considered is the relationship between screening and prevention. Health screening aims to identify risk factors for an illness as primary prevention, early signs, or presymptomatic stages of a disease as secondary prevention, and factors that may modulate the development of disease as tertiary prevention [10]. From such a perspective, screening for complexity fits the criteria of tertiary prevention, because its main purpose is to prevent negative effects on quality of life and outcomes of care. When complexity becomes a more integrated concept in the practice of health care, however, complexity screening might expand to other levels of prevention. Secondary prevention, for example, could also be operationalized in terms of early signs and presymptomatic stages of complexity. For instance, early signs of noncompliance in patients who have diabetes as demonstrated by HbA1c levels, could be an early identifier of complexity. Missed or excessive visits or hospital admissions or excessive use, such as repeated consultations for unexplained physical complaints, could become identifiers for secondary prevention of depression and somatization.

From traditional to integrated care

When a physician encounters a patient who has a clinical problem that does not belong to his area of expertise, and action seems appropriate, the standard medical procedure is to consult a colleague. The authors, however, have demonstrated that such classic ad hoc models are not very effective in identifying and treating certain patients (eg, those who have psychiatric morbidity in the general hospital). Consultations generally are limited compared with the prevalence of a given problem (eg, frailty or psychiatric morbidity) and are initiated much too late in the course of disease (see also the article by Wulsin and colleagues in this issue) [11–13]. The same problems exist in the integration of geriatric care in general practice. This problem was addressed recently in a *Statement of Principles: Toward Improved Care of Older Patients in Surgical and Medical Specialties* by the Interdisciplinary Leadership Group of the American Geriatric Society Project to Increase Geriatric Expertise in Surgical and Medical Specialties [14,15]. The concept of chronic disease management represents an important shift from the traditional consultation model. In these programs epidemiologic knowledge related to a specific disease is taken into account and converted into multidisciplinary protocolized management programs [16]. Such programs have secondary preventive purposes, that is, to detect early signs or presymptomatic stages of possible complications of the disease. In a recent editorial in the *British Medical Journal* Wagner [17] stated that managed-care organizations that use explicit models and strategies for improving care, generally (1) promote self-management by patients, as well as structured visits and follow-up, (2) provide clinical case management of the more complex patients, and (3) improve their decision-support and clinical information systems. Disease-management programs always consist of multidisciplinary teams, which might include nurse case managers, medical specialists, clinical pharmacists, social workers, and sometimes lay health workers.

Historically, first disease management programs, the depression-management programs were initiated by the National Institute of Mental Health Depression Awareness, Recognition and Treatment Program, launched in 1988 [18]. It led to two major branches, one for the management of depression in primary care, and the other for the management of depression in the general hospital led by consultation-liaison psychiatry, or psychosomatic medicine, the new subspecialty of psychiatry in the medically ill [19]. Examples of implementations are programs for the management of physical symptoms (see the article by Kroenke and Rosmalen in this issue), the diabetes depression programs (see the article by Egede and colleagues in this issue), and the Improving Mood—Promoting Access to Collaborative Treatment (IMPACT), a geriatric depression program in primary care [20–22]. The integration of mental health care in these programs is based on the Patient Health Questionnaire 9 (PHQ-9) (Fig. 3) [23], which is discussed below.

Disease-specific versus complexity-specific approaches

The PHQ is a self-reported questionnaire derived from the psychiatric diagnostic tool for primary care, the Primary Care Evaluation of Mental Disorders, based on the *Diagnostic and Statistical Manual of Mental Disorders* [24]. The PHQ is used as a tool to determine action (Box 1), a major advantage of disease-management programs as compared with the traditional consultation model.

PHQ - 9

1. Over the <u>last 2 weeks</u>, how often have you been bothered by the following problems?	Not at all 0	Several days 1	More than half the days 2	Nearly every day 3
a. Little interest or pleasure in doing things	☐	☐	☐	☑
b. Feeling down, depressed, or hopeless	☐	☑	☐	☐
c. Trouble falling or staying asleep, or sleeping too much	☐	☐	☑	☐
d. Feeling tired or having little energy	☐	☐	☐	☑
e. Poor appetite or overeating	☐	☑	☐	☐
f. Feeling bad about yourself, or that you are a failure . . .	☐	☐	☑	☐
g. Trouble concentrating on things, such as reading . . .	☐	☐	☐	☑
h. Moving or speaking so slowly . . .	☑	☐	☐	☐
i. Thoughts that you would be better off dead . . .	☐	☑	☐	☐
Subtotals:		3	4	9

TOTAL = 16

Fig. 3. Patient Health Questionnaire-9. (*Adapted from* PRIME MD TODAY, developed by Drs. Robert L. Spitzer, Janet B.W. Williams, Kurt Kroenke, and colleagues, with an educational grant from Pfizer Inc. For research information, contact Dr. Spitzer at rls8@columbia.edu. Copyright © 1999 Pfizer Inc., used with permission.)

The question arises: should identifiers be disease-specific—as with the PHQ for depression—or focus on behaviors that lead to negative outcomes, such as noncompliance or inadequate health care use? In other words should the identifier be disease specific or complexity specific? For a given disease-management program, such as for diabetes or chronic heart failure, where the prevalence and negative impact of depression are known, disease-specific screening for depression may be appropriate to identify complex patients in need of integrated care. Complexity assessment focusing not only on mood but all kinds of risks associated with chronic diseases, on the other hand, might allow the initiation of comprehensive care and improve outcome and cost effectiveness for a broader group of patients. Further research is needed to determine which approach, disease-specific or complexity-specific, is most appropriate for a given population.

This issue will become more apparent when looking at the role of the nurse practitioners in the Pathway and IMPACT studies [20,21,25]. Because

---

Box 1. Translating PHQ-9 scores into action

0–4 No action (community screens)
5–9 Watchful waiting in most
10–14 Education; counseling; active drug prescription based
    upon diagnosis, duration, impairment, and patient preferences
20+ May need combined medication and/or referral

the primary focus of the Pathway program was to intervene in depression, most nurses involved in the program were specially trained mental health nurses. Cora Hartwell, one of the nurses who was professionally dual trained, saw the need for a broad spectrum of roles requiring differing clinical skills, such as diagnosing depressed patients; educating them about depression and antidepressant medications; encouraging adherence to treatment for depression and also for the physical disorders; dealing with medication side effects; providing brief, structured counseling; organizing patient referral when needed and coordinating care with primary care providers; consulting psychiatrists; and maintaining relapse prevention (personal communication, October 2005).

The IMPACT and related studies illustrate the tensions involved in the use of a disease-specific instead of a generic complexity-specific focus. The possible superiority of a complexity-specific approach is illustrated by the fact that, on average, patients had 3.8 chronic conditions in addition to the depression. More than 50% of these patients suffered from high blood pressure, arthritis, loss of hearing or vision, or chronic pain. Thirty percent had heart disease (angina, failure, valve problems), and between 20% and 25% had asthma, chronic bronchitis or emphysema, or diabetes [20,21]. These comorbidities, as well as social comorbidities, interfere with the treatment of depression, for example, with regard to the adjustment of antidepressants to the needs of the physical morbidities, the compliance management or to the social situation of the patients. Current epidemiologic findings report that about 40% to 50% of patients who have chronic conditions have multiple chronic conditions. This finding suggests that in such disease-management programs patients also have to deal with the complications of cardiovascular-related disease and in later phases of the illness with cognitive decline. Moreover, the problem of comorbidity among psychiatric diagnoses is widely accepted as a major problem of current psychiatric diagnostic systems (see the article by Kroenke and Rosmalen in this issue). Under a disease-specific management program in clinical practice, such patients would require separate care managers for diabetes, cardiac disease, depression, and anxiety or cognition difficulties! Here the issue is to differentiate between patients requiring classic disease management and those who need adjusted, coordinated care because their problems are too complex for a disease-management program focusing on depression care only. Because research has shown that depression is related to increased health care use and noncompliance (see the article by Egede in this issue), one might decide to integrate additional identifiers, such as excessive use, number of missed visits, repeated HbA1c levels beyond 7 or 8 mmol/L, or the number of medical specialists seen [26]. A complexity assessment might, therefore, be more appropriate in this population. Another advantage of the complexity assessment in comparison with a depression screener is that the former provides a broader insight in the health risks of a given patient and also detects actions that should be taken.

Identifiers of complex medically ill patients

The foregoing discussion indicates that medical teams should determine identifiers of their complex patients derived from the clinical characteristics of the population they serve. They should use their existing administrative and clinical monitoring system to provide "red flags" as identifiers of complex patients. Such identifiers would be (1) clinical characteristics, such as negative medical outcomes (eg, HbA1c levels in diabetes) or complications (eg, kidney disease in cardiovascular disease) and (2) characteristics of service delivery, such as excessive use, missed appointments or refills, emergency medical admissions, or number of medical specialists other than primary health care providers involved [27]. Populations also can qualify for a need for integrated

---

Box 2. Identifiers of complexity

Clinical identifiers of complexity
Illness
   Disease (stage)
   Clinical parameters
   Negative health behavior
   Noncompliance
   Persisting unexplained physical complaints (see also
      Kroenke and Rosmalen, Table 2)
Highly intensive and demanding treatments
   Intensive cancer treatment
   Hemodialysis
   Transplantation
Organization of care
   Number of participating health care professionals and
      institutions
   Health care use (missed or excessive)
   Conflicts/miscommunication
Instruments to assess complexity
   Complexity Prediction Instrument (COMPRI) (see also
      de Jonge and colleagues in this issue)
   Groningen Frailty Index (see Slaets in this issue)
   The INTERMED method (see Stiefel and colleagues in this
      issue)
Clinimetric
   Patient Health Questionnaire 9 (see also Kroenke and
      Rosmalen in this issue)
   Patient Health Questionnaire 2 [28]
   Distress thermometer [29]

care by the origin of their illness (eg, hepatitis C due to high risk behavior), symptoms (eg, unexplained physical complaints), or the complexity of the required treatment and the related distress produced (eg, transplantation). A list of possible identifiers of complexity is provided in Box 2. As mentioned in the Preface to this issue, identification of complexity must be followed by an adequate assessment that provides useful clinical information required for an integrated treatment plan. Only a few instruments have been designed to detect or assess complexity. The INTERMED method, discussed in detail in the article by Stiefel and colleagues in this issue, is such an instrument [6,7]. It is empirically based and has been evaluated with regard to reliability, validity, and predictive validity. The INTERMED method is based on the communi-metric approach (see the article by Lyons in this issue). It contains 16 health risks, such as whether a patient has a chronic disease, has had diagnostic problems in the past or currently, is physically impaired, is able to cope, has had psychiatric episodes in the past or has current psychiatric symptoms, complies with treatment, has had negative experiences with health care providers, or demonstrates increased health care use and social difficulties or lack of support. The INTERMED is an action–oriented assessment method for case complexity but can also serve as generic identifiers of complexity in populations that cannot easily be screened by the clinical or service delivery identifiers discussed here. It is especially useful in populations where complex patients are a majority (eg, transplantation, high proportion of somatizers).

References

[1] Huyse FJ, Herzog T, Malt UF, et al. A screening instrument for the detection of psychosocial risk factors in patients admitted to general hospital wards (grant number BMH1–CT93–1180). In: Baert A, et al, editors. Biomedical and health research. The BIOMED1 programme. Bruxelles, Belgium: Ohmsha IOS Press; 1995.

[2] Huyse FJ. From consultation to complexity of care prediction and health service needs assessment [editorial]. J Psychosom Res 1997;43:233–40.

[3] De Jonge P, Huyse FJ, Slaets JP, et al. Care complexity in the general hospital: results from a European study. Psychosomatics 2001a;42(3):204–12.

[4] De Jonge P, Huyse FJ, Herzog T, et al. Risk factors for complex care needs in general medical inpatients: results from a European study. Psychosomatics 2001b;42(3):213–21.

[5] Huyse FJ, de Jonge P, Slaets JP, et al. COMPRI—an instrument to detect patients with complex care needs: results from a European study. Psychosomatics 2001a;42(3):222–8.

[6] Huyse FJ, Lyons JS, Stiefel FC, et al. "INTERMED": a method to assess health service needs: I. Development and reliability. Gen Hosp Psychiatry 1999;21:39–48.

[7] Stiefel FC, de Jonge P, Huyse FJ, et al. "INTERMED": a method to assess health service needs: II. Results on its validity and clinical use. Gen Hosp Psychiatry 1999;21:49–56.

[8] Institute of Medicine. Crossing the quality chasm: a new health system for the 21st century. Committee on Quality of Health Care in America. Washington (DC): National Academy Press; 2001.

[9] Trzepacz P, Dimartini A. The transplant patient. Biological, psychiatric and ethical issues in organ transplantation. Cambridge (UK): Cambridge University Press; 2000.

[10] Rimes K, Salkovskis P. Health screening programs. In: Gelder MG, Lòpez-Ibor JJ, Andreasen NC, editors. The new Oxford textbook of psychiatry. New York: Oxford University Press; 2000.

[11] Huyse FJ, Herzog T, Lobo A, et al. European consultation-liaison services and their user populations: the European Consultation-Liaison Workgroup Collaborative Study. Psychosomatics 2000;41(4):330–8.

[12] Huyse FJ, Herzog T, Lobo A, et al. Consultation-liaison psychiatric service delivery: results from a European study. Gen Hosp Psychiatry 2001b;23(3):124–32.

[13] Wallen J, Pincus HA, Goldman HH, et al. Psychiatric consultation in short-term general hospitals. Arch Gen Psychiatry 1987;44(2):163–8.

[14] Interdisciplinary Leadership Group of the American Geriatric Society Project to Increase Geriatric Expertise in Surgical and Medical Specialties. A statement of principles: towards improved care of older patients in surgical and medical specialties. J Am Geriatr Soc 2000;48:699–701.

[15] Solomon DH, Burton JR, Lundebjerg, et al. The new frontier: increasing geriatric expertise in surgical and medical specialties. J Am Geriatr Soc 2000;48:702–4.

[16] Wagner EH. Chronic disease care. BMJ 2004;328:177–8.

[17] Wagner EH. The role of patient care teams in chronic disease management. BMJ 2000;320: 569–72.

[18] Regier DA, Hirschfeld RM, Goodwin FK, et al. The NIMH depression awareness, recognition, and treatment program. Am J Psychiatry 1988;145(11):1351–7.

[19] Gitlin DF, Levenson JL, Lyketsos CG. Psychosomatic medicine: a new medical subspecialty. Acad Psychiatry 2004;28(1):4–11.

[20] Unutzer J, Katon W, Williams JW, et al. Improving primary care for depression in late life; the design of a multicenter randomized trial. Med Care 2001;39(8):785–99.

[21] Unutzer J, Katon W, Callahan CM, et al. Collaborative care management of late-life depression in the primary care setting: a randomized controlled trial. JAMA 2002;288(22):2836–45.

[22] Harpole LH, Williams JW, Olsen MK, et al. Improving depression outcomes in older adults with co-morbid medical illness. Gen Hosp Psychiatry 2005;27(1):4–12.

[23] Kroenke K, Spitzer RL, Williams JBW. The PHQ-9; validity of a brief depression severity measure. J Gen Intern Med 2001;16:606–13.

[24] Spitzer RL, Kroenke K, Willaims JB. Validation and utility of a self report version of the PRIME-MD; the PHQ primary care study. Primary Care Evaluation of Mental Disorders. Patient Health Questionnaire. JAMA 1999;282(18):1737–44.

[25] Katon WJ, Von Korff M, Lin EH, et al. The Pathways study: a randomized trial of collaborative care in patients with diabetes and depression. Arch Gen Psychiatry 2004;61: 1042–9.

[26] Fischer CJ, Stiefel FC, De Jonge P, et al. Case complexity and clinical outcome in diabetes mellitus. A prospective study using the INTERMED. Diabetes Metab 2000;26(4):295–302.

[27] Shea S, DuMouchel W, Bahamonde L. A meta-analysis of 16 randomized controlled trials to evaluate computer-based clinical reminder systems for preventive care in the ambulatory setting. JAMA 1996;3:399–409.

[28] Kroenke K, Spitzer RL, Williams JB. The Patient Health Questionnaire-2: validity of a two-item depression screener. Med Care 2003;41(11):1284–9.

[29] Jacobson PB, Donovan KA, Trask PC, et al. Screening for psychological distress in ambulatory cancer patients. Cancer 2005;103(7):1494–502.

ELSEVIER
SAUNDERS

Med Clin N Am 90 (2006) 713–758

THE MEDICAL
CLINICS
OF NORTH AMERICA

Operationalizing Integrated Care on a Clinical Level: the INTERMED Project

Friedrich C. Stiefel, MD, PhD[a],*,
Frits J. Huyse, MD, PhD[b], Wolfgang Söllner, MD[c],
Joris P.J. Slaets, MD, PhD[b], John S. Lyons, PhD[d],
Corine H.M. Latour, CNS, RN[e],
Nynke van der Wal, ANP[b], Peter de Jonge, PhD[b,f]

[a]Service de Psychiatrie de Liaison, Centre Hospitalier
Universitaire Vaudois, Rue du Bugnon 44, CH-1011 Lausanne, Switzerland
[b]Department of General Internal Medicine, University Medical Center Groningen,
Hanzeplein 1, 9700 RB, Groningen, The Netherlands
[c]General Hospital Nuremberg, Prof. Ernst-Nathan-Strasse 1, 90419 Nürnberg, Germany
[d]Feinberg School of Medicine, Northwestern University,
Weibolt 717, 339 East Chicago Avenue, Chicago, IL 60611, USA
[e]Psychiatric Consultation and Liaison Service, Vrije Universiteit University Medical Center,
De Boelelaan 1117 1081HV Amsterdam, The Netherlands
[f]Department of Psychiatry, University of Groningen, Hanzeplein 1,
Gebouw 32 9700 RB, Groningen, The Netherlands

Other articles in this issue present relevant arguments why assessment and treatment of psychosocial comorbidities should be integrated in the provision of general medical care. Psychosocial comorbidities, highly prevalent because of an increase in numbers of the elderly and of patients who have chronic diseases [1], influence the outcome of various somatic diseases [2] and are associated with excessive health care use [3], diminished quality of life [4], survival [5], and compliance with treatments, which represents a major obstacle to effective medical care [6]. Moreover, several symptoms co-occur in psychiatric and somatic syndromes; for example, some psychiatric disorders such as depression have somatic symptoms [7], and physiologic and behavioral mechanisms have been described that cross the borders between somatic and psychiatric disciplines, such as in depression and coronary

---

* Corresponding author.
E-mail address: frederic.stiefel@chuv.ch (F.C. Stiefel).

0025-7125/06/$ - see front matter © 2006 Elsevier Inc. All rights reserved.
doi:10.1016/j.mcna.2006.05.006   *medical.theclinics.com*

artery disease and diabetes mellitus (see articles in this issue by Kroenke and Rosmalen and by Egede). Finally, many risk factors for somatic and psychiatric diseases are shared, for example in the concept of frailty or in the metabolic syndrome (see articles in this issue by Slaets and by Gans).

Despite these arguments, the biopsychosocial model of disease [8] has not been implemented in standard general health care, resulting in undertreatment of psychiatric and psychosocial comorbidities [9,10]. Although several attempts have been made to operationalize the biopsychosocial model of disease and to develop related assessment instruments, efficient methods for use in general clinical care are still lacking [11,12]. The issue of how to approach biopsychosocial morbidity thus remains an important challenge. This article describes the INTERMED project, which aims to operationalize the biopsychosocial model of disease and to fill the gap between general medical and mental health care. The INTERMED is an interview-based instrument to assess case complexity and allows a quick evaluation of biopsychosocial health risks and the related treatment planning [13–15].

The INTERMED method: operationalizing the biopsychosocial model of disease

The INTERMED project was initiated to develop an instrument to assess biopsychosocial case complexity (see the article in this issue by de Jonge and colleagues). In contrast to the patient-grouping methodologies, the INTERMED was not designed to collect diagnostic data, because such data often are not available at the beginning of the process of care delivery and often explain only a limited amount of the variance with regard to health care use. Also, in contrast to other methodologies assessing complexity, the INTERMED could not rely on existing data, because many of the relevant psychosocial patient characteristics are not routinely collected in general health care. To start developing a method to assess biopsychosocial case complexity and to define related integrated treatment plans, the authors therefore first relied on clinical experience with the format of life charts, as introduced by Querido [16], and on similar approaches (Fig. 1) [11,17].

This format has been used for many years to analyze and supervise complex medical cases in multidisciplinary conferences by drawing the patient's situation on white boards (Fig. 2). The life chart offers a structured approach to organize clinical data with regard to biologic, psychologic, social, and health care–related aspects in a context of time. As such, the life chart provides an opportunity to develop an integrated treatment plan.

Based on clinical experience with the life chart and epidemiologic literature on characteristics influencing patients' treatment response and health care use, a first pool of variables was selected to develop the INTERMED. In 1995 the communimetric approach for assessment instruments for the mental health field was introduced (see the article in this issue by Lyons [18]), and a first version of the INTERMED was integrated in a research

Examples of life charts

Querido [16]	Physical Factors	Psychologic Factors	Social Factors
Time-axis↓			
Nurcombe-Gallagher [17]	Predisposing Factors	Precipitating Factors	Maintaining Factors
Biologic			
Psychologic			
Social system			
Health care system			
Leigh [11]	Current State	Recent Events	Background
Biologic			
Psychologic			
Social system			
Health care system			

Fig. 1. Systems of life charts. (*Data from* Refs. [11,16,17]).

project granted by the European Union for the European Consultation-Liaison Workgroup [19]. The main objective of this project was to develop an instrument to detect patients who had complex care needs; the development of the Complexity Prediction Instrument (COMPRI) assessment was derived from this project [20]. Thereafter, an international multidisciplinary group consisting of consultation-liaison psychiatrists, psychologists, and colleagues from different somatic disciplines continued to elaborate the INTERMED. This process resulted in the grid and the variables shown in Table 1.

The INTERMED describes the biologic, psychologic, social, and health care characteristics of the patient in a time perspective consisting of his

	Facts Time-axis ⟶	Interventions
Bio		
Psy		
Soc		
HC		

Fig. 2. Structured life chart for organizing clinical data.

Table 1
Variables of the INTERMED schema

Domain	History	Current State	Prognoses
Biologic	Chronicity	Severity of symptoms	Complications and life threat
	Diagnostic dilemma	Diagnostic challenge	
Psychologic	Restrictions in coping Psychiatric dysfunctioning	Resistance to treatment Psychiatric symptoms	Mental health threat
Social	Restrictions in integration	Residential instability	Social vulnerability
	Social dysfunctioning	Restrictions of network	
Health care	Intensity of treatment Treatment experience	Organization of care Appropriateness of referral	Coordination

From: Huyse FJ, Lyons JS, Stiefel FC, et al. "INTERMED": a method to assess health service needs: I. Development and reliability. Gen Hosp Psychiatry 1999;21:41.

history, current state, and prognoses. The INTERMED is structured in 12 cells to organize information. Two pertinent variables were selected from the variable pool for each cell of the History and Current State columns, and one variable was selected for each cell of the Prognoses column. The selection of these 20 variables was discussed and validated (face validity) by a panel of researchers and clinicians.

Description of the INTERMED

The material presented in the articles in this issue provides the knowledge base on which the INTERMED was constructed. The reader is referred to these articles. A few additional references are provided here.

History

Biologic domain

In the "History" biologic domain information is collected about the chronicity of a given illness ("Chronicity") and about prior episodes of diagnostic uncertainty ("Diagnostic dilemma"). The distinction between acute and chronic diseases has proven helpful for the conceptualization of somatic diseases and the patient's care needs, especially in the elderly. It also is an indicator for the risk of a comorbid psychiatric disturbance, because the prevalence of psychiatric disturbances is increased in chronic medical illnesses (see also articles in this issue by Kathol and colleagues and by Slaets and [21,22]). Diagnostic uncertainty, especially when reflected in multiple testing and contradictory medical diagnoses, indicates possible episodes of depressive, anxiety-related, or somatoform disorders, which are known to increase case complexity and health care use and to diminish response to medical treatments or the existence of a rare or complex physical disease (see also articles in this issue by Kathol and colleagues and by Kroenke and Rosmalen and [23,24]).

Psychologic domain

In the "History" psychologic domain information is collected about past coping resources ("Restrictions in coping") and psychiatric history ("Psychiatric dysfunctioning"). Both are known to increase case complexity and health care use, to diminish treatment response, and to enlarge the expression of functional physical symptoms. As a result, patients who have such disturbances have increased health care needs (see also articles in this issue by Kathol and colleagues and by Kroenke and Rosmalen and [21,25–27]). Because psychiatric morbidity has a tendency to become chronic, the two variables are predictive for the patient's current and future adaptation to the disease and therefore for prospective care needs. In contrast to the other variables, which are assessed over the last 5 years, the variable "Psychiatric dysfunctioning" is assessed as a lifetime variable, because it is known that psychiatric disorders—even those that occurred many years ago—can reflect psychiatric vulnerability when facing current medical stressors [21].

Social domain

In the "History" social domain information is collected about social integration in terms of having a job and leisure activities ("Restrictions of integration") and the patient's capacity to maintain relations ("Social dysfunctioning"). Being socially embedded has been proven to influence adaptation to somatic illness; this domain thus reflects the patient's social needs. Moreover, it has been demonstrated that social isolation is associated with an impaired prognosis of somatic illnesses, such as cardiovascular disease [28,29].

Health care domain

In the "History" health care domain information is collected about intensity ("Intensity") and adequacy of prior care ("Treatment experience"). Health care use during prior episodes of illness and the quality of past relationships with health care providers are likely to influence current and future care needs. Patients who have had negative experiences, such as missed medical diagnoses or conflicts with staff, are likely to be suspicious or distrustful in future relations with clinicians and therefore may be seek unnecessary second opinions and engage in doctor-shopping (see also the article in this issue by Kathol and colleagues and [30]).

Current state

Biologic domain

In the "Current State" biologic domain information is collected about the severity of physical symptoms and related physical impairment

("Severity of symptoms"), as well as about complexity of the medical diagnosis ("Diagnostic challenge"). Both variables are related to current therapeutic medical/nursing needs (see articles in this issue by Kathol and colleagues, by Kroenke and Rosmalen, and by Egede and [31]).

Psychologic domain

In the "Current State" psychologic domain information is collected about the level of cooperation of the patient with the recommended treatment ("Resistance to treatment") and current psychiatric disturbances ("Psychiatric symptoms"). Compliance and psychiatric comorbidity, such as cognitive impairment, substance abuse, and depression, are interrelated and are crucial for the outcome of medical illness (see the article in this issue by Egede and [21,32]).

Social domain

In the "Current State" social domain information is collected about patients' current living situation ("Residential instability") and supportive social relations, such as family, friends, or colleagues ("Restrictions of network"). These variables influence adjustment to disease and the organization of care [28,29].

Health care domain

In the "Current State" health care domain information is collected about the organizational complexity in terms of number and types of health care providers involved in the care before referral or admission ("Organization of care"). This information reflects both the intensity and complexity of the care that will have to be delivered. Here also the appropriateness of transitions of care such as referral and hospitalization is evaluated ("Appropriateness of referral"). These variables assess the complexity of care and the possible divisions and fragmentations within the system (ie, primary care versus secondary care or general care versus mental health care) that might have negative effects on care [33].

Prognosis

Biologic domain

In the "Prognosis" biologic domain information is collected about the anticipated outcomes of the disease, such as impairments, complications, or recurrence of disease or life threat. All of these outcomes are of major importance for the future medical needs of a patient and related treatment planning.

Psychologic domain

In the "Prognosis" psychologic domain information is collected about the anticipated mental health threat and related psychologic needs that may result from the current illness episode or past psychiatric history.

Social domain

In the "Prognosis" social domain information is collected about the anticipated social needs with regard to the social integration of the patient. This information is most important for those patients who have had changes in their physical and psychologic status resulting in social disintegration, such as physical dependence or social isolation, which might require adjustment of care (ie, provision of additional support at home or temporary admission to a facility) [28].

Health care domain

In the "Prognosis" health care domain information is collected about anticipated health care needs in terms of intensity and the complexity of its organization. The health service needs on the different system levels (biologic, psychologic, and social) are accumulated and, depending on their mutual interference, the need to integrate health services is evaluated. Additional efforts may be needed to organize care, for example, through multidisciplinary case conferences (horizontal coordination of care) or initiation and monitoring of longitudinal care trajectories by a case manager (vertical coordination of care).

Scoring of the INTERMED

In another article in this issue, Lyons describes a communimetric approach to develop action-oriented clinical decision-support systems, specifically for the management of patients who have complex needs and who are cared for in complex medical systems. In this scenario appropriate and efficient communication among health professionals becomes crucial. In contrast to psychometric methods, which were developed for research and have limited meaning for clinical work, communimetric assessment instruments are action oriented and geared toward clinical decision making and management. The mixed psychometric, clinimetric, and communimetric approach (see articles in this issue by de Jonge and colleagues, by Lyons, and by Huyse and colleagues and the section on the scientific evaluation of the INTERMED in this article) in developing the INTERMED resulted in an action-oriented decision-support tool for the management of complex medical cases. The universal scoring and the use of uniform colors (green, yellow, orange, and red) of the variables to indicate risks and needs for actions facilitate the integration of the INTERMED in clinical practice (Fig. 3) [15].

For each variable, specific clinical anchor points were defined to facilitate reliable scoring. The scores on the variables can be summed to a total score ranging from 0 to 60, reflecting the level of complexity of the case (see Appendix 1).

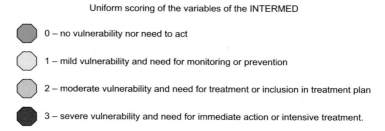

Fig. 3. Uniform scoring of the variables of the INTERMED. (*Adapted from* Huyse FJ, Lyons JS, Stiefel FC, et al. Operationalizing the biopsychosocial model. The INTERMED [editorial]. Psychosomatics 2001;42(1):5–13.)

Data collection and clinical interview

Data collection with the INTERMED depends on the profession of the assigned user and the setting. For example, a trained physician is able to conduct the full interview and obtain scoring, whereas a trained nurse will be able to assess almost all variables with the exception of the variables "Diagnostic challenge" and the "Biological prognosis," for which the treating physician must be consulted. When used in an outpatient setting for selected cases identified by "red flags" or identifiers (see the article in this issue by Huyse and colleagures), a separate appointment for an assessment can be made with the patient.

The patient is guided through the different domains in a coherent and emotionally acceptable and supportive way. This approach is crucial to establish a relationship and foster mutual understanding of the problems to be faced. Thirteen leading questions help ensure that the patient provides the relevant information (see Appendix 2). The sequence of the 13 questions is not absolute; once familiar with the INTERMED interview, raters can use their own style and adjust the sequence to the specific information provided by the patient [15].

Before the interview, the clinician should evaluate existing information by reviewing the patient's medical history, the reason for referral or admission, and relevant psychosocial information. When starting the interview, the clinician may use a short introduction, such as:

> Now that we know about your medical situation, I would like to get a better idea what kind of person you are and how are you dealing with your medical problems; this information will help organize medical care tailored to your specific individual needs. Because we have to discuss several issues, I might interrupt you sometimes when I feel that I know enough for a comprehensive overview of your problems.

After covering the biologic domains, a summary of the available information is provided, and the patient is asked if this information seems appropriate from his or her perspective. Subsequently the specific information concerning the health care domains is collected; then a shift is made toward the social domains, and, finally, the variables of the psychologic domains are explored. At the end of the interview the interviewer underlines the importance of the information provided by the patient and summarizes and verifies the most relevant information. Then the interviewer asks whether pertinent issues have been missed and invites the patient to express how he or she felt about the interview. Finally the patient is informed how the information will be handled and the next steps he or she can expect. The authors' clinical experience is that almost all medical patients are satisfied with the interview, with the occasional exception of patients who have severe somatization, who may feel threatened by questions concerning their psychologic state. The authors often have heard patients say, "You are the first clinician who is not only interested in my disease, but also in me as a person who has to deal with the illness." With regard to the question whether pertinent issues have been missed, most patients do not think so. An as yet unpublished scientific evaluation of patients has demonstrated that patients generally are very satisfied with the INTERMED interview.

The INTERMED interview in specific patient populations

For elderly patients or in patients who have indications of cognitive disturbances, a series of questions is asked to evaluate cognitive impairment. Such questions derived from cognitive screening tests could be: "Can you tell me why you are here?" If not: "Can you tell me what kind of person I am?", "Can you tell me where you are?", or "Can you tell me what date it is?" In case of incorrect answers, one might decide to interview a partner or someone else close to the patient, including professionals who care or cared for the patient.

For patients who are very anxious, depressed, or emotionally disturbed one might consider asking a consultation-liaison psychiatrist, a psychologist, or a psychiatric nurse to conduct the interview, or it might be important to wait until the patient agrees to provide information about sensitive issues such as social integration. It is especially important to obtain such information from these patients, because the information is most likely to influence the current illness episode.

Patients suffering from severe somatization may be reluctant to provide information about their psychologic state and the history of their social integration; this reluctance may result from alexithymia or a fear that their symptoms may be linked to psychologic factors and not be taken seriously by the clinician. If patients cannot be assured that their symptoms are taken seriously or if they seem unable to express their emotional state, the lacking information in the INTERMED grid should alert the clinician to reflect on the case and to consider a psychiatric disturbance, such as somatization.

In the following section a case is presented in all its details, from available information, through the interview and the process of scoring, followed by the organization of the written information and a plan for treatment [15]. Appendix 3 presents additional cases that can be used for scoring.

Example of an INTERMED interview: the case of Mr. Glover

Information available at admission: Mr. Glover is a 55-year-old married real estate salesman who comes to the emergency room after having been pressured by an employee of his firm to consult a physician. He has symptoms indicating a possible myocardial infarction; he already has been hospitalized for a first myocardial infarction 6 months earlier. The investigations in the emergency room confirm the diagnosis. While in the emergency room the patient develops ventricular fibrillation requiring cardioversion, sedation, and admission. The patient is admitted to a cardiology ward where an emergency admission is a indicator ("red flag") for an INTERMED assessment.

A trained nurse conducts the interview on the next day, after the patient is physically stabilized and has had some rest. The cardiologist informs the nurse about the diagnosis and physical status. The diagnosis is a second myocardial infarction of a person known to have arterial hypertension without evident signs of pump failure. The patient, whose circulation has been stabilized after the cardioversion, is confined to his bed and will later have a cardiac work-up. According to the protocol, the cardiac work-up requires standard cardiology follow-up and a postdischarge rehabilitation program. It is expected that the patient will be slightly limited in his physical activities (New York Heart Association classification 1–2). Mr. Glover, who has not seen his wife in the last months, asks only that his sister be informed about his condition. The sister seems very concerned when she hears what happened, and she announces to the nurse that she will visit Mr. Glover the next day.

After a stable night during which the patient slept well with hypnotics, the nurse starts the INTERMED interview. She begins with the following opening question: "I heard you have been admitted for a myocardial infarction and that your situation has stabilized since yesterday. To be able to provide the best treatment, we would like to know a little bit more about who you are and how it is for you to be here. Now, first of all, how do you feel physically"?

The patient reports that he does not have pain or other physical complaints. He knows he did not feel well the day before. He remembers having visited the emergency room and that the doctor informed him that he had suffered a myocardial event, but he still cannot believe it. He thought the physical symptoms he experienced before admission were related to a bad night of sleep. The nurse informs Mr. Glover that although he is currently stable, he must stay in bed for a while. She then states, "I will tell you what I know about the reason for your admission and your current state. You should correct me when I am wrong," and provides the information described by the cardiologist. Then she informs him that she would like to know more about the circumstances of this current illness episode: "Now I would like to know how you felt emotionally during the last week"?

Mr. Glover answers that he had been feeling tense; he did not sleep well at all and felt blue during the last weeks. To try to get to sleep and to cheer himself up, he had been drinking several whiskies in the evenings. When asked, he said that he does not feel tense now because of not having alcohol, but he would not mind to have something to smoke. When the nurse asks him whether feeling blue is related to the problems with his wife, the patient confirms her suggestion.

The nurse tells Mr. Glover that this is important information and that she will come back to this issue and then goes on, "I would like to have some more information concerning the physical illnesses and treatments of the past 5 years." Mr. Glovers informs the nurse that he has had a myocardial infarction about 6 months ago for which he was admitted. For more than 15 years he has suffered from uncomplicated hypertension for which he has been taking medication. There has not been any other reason to see a doctor. The nurse then asks "Who are the doctors who have taken care for you in the last 5 years?" A primary care physician had treated the patient's hypertension. After his first cardiac infarction, the patient had seen a cardiologist twice. The cardiologist had pointed to his life-style and suggested to see a psychologist to discuss his attitude toward work. Because he was too busy and was anxious about keeping up with his new job, he did not follow these recommendations. The nurse continues "Have you ever seen a psychiatrist in your life or have there been periods that you have been anxious, depressed, or confused"? Mr. Glover states that he was "depressed" once, a long time ago, when his first wife divorced him. For half a year he became very passive and was not able to work. He consulted a psychiatrist and was treated with antidepressants. He stopped his medication and psychiatric follow-up when he moved to another town. Currently, he does not know, but perhaps he might again be depressed. His new job is stressful, and he is again in conflict and without the support of his wife; living in a hotel room for the past few weeks has been tough. The nurse emphasizes the importance of this information. She says that she will come back to this issue.

Then she continues and asks the patient to specify. "Now who are the doctors, nurses, social workers or psychologists who are currently taking care for you"? Mr. Glover answers that there has been no time for consultations; the last time had been tense and busy. He should have seen his cardiologist but failed to do so. Maybe he should have seen a psychologist, too, he says. To the nurse's question "Have there been issues with doctors during the last 5 years that gave you a bad feeling to the extent that it might interfere with your trust in doctors?" Mr. Glover replies that at the end of his previous cardiac admission the patient next to him died unexpectedly during the night. Afterwards he heard that the hospital had organizational problems for which it had been sued. In addition, during his last visit to the cardiologist, when he mentioned that he and his wife were in conflict concerning his current job, the cardiologist did not react and continued to focus on his cardiac condition. These events changed his view towards doctors. "You simply cannot rely on them," he states. The nurse confirms that she thinks this is important information, also, because trust in your doctor is crucial. She continues, "I would like to know how you follow your doctor's recommendations. Are you a person who, generally speaking, is inclined to do what doctors say?" Mr. Glover answers that concerning his medication, for years he has been a regular user. During the last month it was a mess, it was impossible to keep up with the regimen.

"Now I would like to change the subject and ask you how you currently live," the nurse states. The patient reports that his wife did not want to follow him to the new job. There had been quarrels concerning the interference of his work with the marriage. When Mr. Glover insisted on changing his job and moving, his wife said that she did not want to see him for a while. This happened about 1 month ago. Consequently, he was living in a hotel room and looking for an apartment. He meets with a colleague once a week; otherwise, he works late and eats in restaurants. The nurse confirms that she sees the problem and continues: "Now I would like to know what kind of person you are. Generally speaking, are you an easygoing person"? The patient replies that his wife would say that he is a difficult person to live with, but he does not think so. He does not need many people as long as he can work. For him, it is important to be successful, and "That's not an easy job." In recent weeks he had felt that he was not fully in control of the situation. The nurse asked him whether everything was an effort and whether he felt blue or hopeless about the future, and the patient confirmed that he did. Mr. Glover ignored her question as to whether he had given up or wanted to die, and he seemed somewhat distressed.

The nurse tells Mr. Glover that, after discussion with the cardiologist, she will consider appropriate consultation and will confirm such consultation soon after the interview. The nurse continues, "Now, coming to the end of the interview, I would like to ask you about your smoking and drinking habits and their relation to the current problems." The patient informs her that he has been drinking up to six whiskies an evening in the last month. He has had earlier periods of heavy drinking. In such periods he smoked, also; lately he smokes only cigars. When asked, he tells the nurse that he never suffered from symptoms of withdrawal. The nurse thanks the patient for all the relevant information he has provided in such a short time. She emphasizes that she understands that he has had a difficult time, that he did not function well, and that this situation will be taken into consideration in the treatment plan. The patient ignores the question, "Do you think we missed any pertinent information?", and the nurse continues, "I finally would like to know how you have experienced this interview? Do you think that this will be helpful information or did you think this was inappropriate?" The patient replies that he feels somewhat relieved and thought the questions were appropriate and helpful.

These guiding questions allow the interviewer to develop the relationship with the patient. The issues progress from medical to more personal matters. The more internalized the interview becomes, and the more skilled the interviewer is, the easier it is to develop a personal interviewing style. Therefore it is most helpful to visualize the schema with the variables, to be able to scan it mentally during the interview for completeness of information. On wards where the method has been implemented, the variables have been integrated in the existing nurse chart based on nurse processing techniques for treatment planning [34].

Scoring of the Glover case

Scoring of the variables is based on matching the clinical data with the clinical anchor points described in Appendix 1. If the clinical information concerning a specific variable does not match the information provided by the anchor points exactly, or in the case of doubts, the rater estimates by comparison with the anchor points how the given information influences the complexity of the patient and the need of action. Here the scoring of the case of Mr. Glover is described; the anchor points referred to in the text are described in Appendix 1. The goal of this scoring example is not to discuss all reflections concerning different scoring options but to provide the reader with an indication of how the INTERMED works and how Mr. Glover would be scored.

1. Chronicity is scored as 3, because the hypertension and the myocardial infarction are seen as two separate medical diagnoses. Although one could argue that the patient has two expressions of the same illness, with the myocardial infarction being a complication of the hypertension, both conditions are chronic, and the prognosis of the combination is worse than that of hypertension alone. Therefore this patient is more complex, as reflected in the highest score on this item.
2. Diagnostic dilemma is scored as a 1, because about half a year ago the patient had a myocardial infarction for which the diagnosis was immediately obtained.
3. Severity of symptoms is scored as 2. In Mr. Glover's case, it is not the patient who provides information on the severity of symptoms and the related functional capacity. Even if he were able to walk around, the cardiologist has decided that he must stay in bed for the first days after his admission and that he is not allowed to perform any functional activities. He therefore scores 2. In most other cases, this item is scored on the basis of the information provided by the patient. For example, a patient who is a severe somatizer would be scored as 2 (ie, having "moderate to severe symptoms that interfere with current functioning").
4. Diagnostic challenge is scored as 0, because the findings are without doubt consistent with a myocardial infarction. If this patient had been diagnosed as not having had an infarction, and the pain was considered

possibly related to anxiety, this variable would have been scored as a 3 (ie, a "complex differential diagnosis, in which no diagnosis is to be expected from a biologic perspective").

5. Restrictions in coping is scored as 2, because the patient has impaired coping skills. Although he has had a serious illness (myocardial infarction) and both his cardiologist and his wife confronted him as being a workaholic, he was not able to face a new job offer adequately, nor had he been able to control his drinking and smoking behavior.

6. Psychiatric dysfunctioning, in contrast to all other variables, is scored from a lifetime perspective. Because the patient once was depressed and unable to function for some time, the score is 2.

7. Resistance to treatment is scored as 2, because the patient did not follow the recommendations provided by the cardiologist, including the suggestion to see a psychologist; in addition, he was not able to follow his medication schedule during the last month. Finally, he was not willing to initiate a medical consultation despite his chest pain and had to be convinced by a colleague to seek medical attention. These serious expressions of noncompliance surpass the anchor point of "some ambivalence, but willing to cooperate with treatment."

8. Psychiatric symptom is scored as 2, because Mr. Glover is not just somewhat tense or has problems in concentrating. There is evidence of significant depressive symptoms. In addition, the patient has a problem with substance abuse (both tobacco and alcohol). Because he shows no symptoms of withdrawal, however, he scores only 2 in this domain.

9. Social integration is scored as 1, because Mr. Glover qualifies as "Having a job without having leisure activities." (Patients who are retired or who do not have a job but who actively take care of their household and patients who are studying are scored as having work.)

10. Social dysfunctioning is scored as 1, because the patient reports quarrels and disagreement with his wife.

11. Residential instability is scored as 3, because the patient has an instable living situation; the score reflects that action is needed. It is assumed, however, that a solution can be found with the help of his sister.

12. Social network is scored as 2, because Mr. Glover has social restrictions in two areas, but he does have a sister and a colleague who are concerned.

13. Intensity of treatment is scored as 2, because the patient was hospitalized about half a year ago. (A score of 3 would be given if the patient had stayed for a longer time on an ICU during his last admission because of serious complications.)

14. Treatment experience (ie, "negative experiences with health care providers [self or relatives]") is scored as 1, because Mr. Glover had mentioned negative perceptions of health care providers on two occasions. A score of 2 (ie, "requests for second opinions or changing contacts with doctors") could be considered, because the patient reported that he had consequently stopped his contact with the cardiologist. This

example shows that the scoring at times may differ slightly between interviewers; still, interrater reliability for the global INTERMED score was always satisfying.

15. Organization of care is scored as 0, because the patient has not been treated by different medical specialists. This variable rates the number of health care providers involved and thereby the potential complexity of communication among care providers. Mr. Glover should have been treated by a cardiologist and a psychologist, but he did not follow these recommendations. The fact that he was not compliant increases his complexity, but this fact has already been reflected in the two variables "Restrictions in coping" and "Resistance to treatment."

16. Appropriateness of admission or referral is scored as 1, because this was an emergency admission ("unplanned referral or admission"). If the patient had been readmitted after a week in a state of self-neglect and heavily drinking, a score of 2 (ie, "able to plan a strategy for treatment, but not able to provide optimal care") would be appropriate.

17. Biologic prognosis is scored as 2, because the patient has a chronic condition or permanent substantial limitations in activities of daily living. For example, if the cardiologist had indicated the myocardial infarction was complicated by a serious risk of dying, a score of 3 would be appropriate.

18. Psychologic prognosis is scored as 2 (ie, "at risk of moderate psychiatric disorder requiring psychiatric care"), because the patient has a current depressive episode, complicated substance abuse, work-related problems, a marital conflict, a serious physical condition, and noncompliance; these associated problems indicate that the depression, as well as the associated psychiatric and psychosocial problems, may persist for quite some time.

19. Social prognosis is scored as 2, because there is a serious risk of a "temporary admission to facility/institution" until a new housing situation can be found with his sister's help.

20. Prognosis of health care: is scored as 3. Because of the various risks in different domains and the high scores with regard to prognoses, Mr. Glover's case requires intensive action, including initiation of a multidisciplinary case conference and long-term coordination of care by a case manager.

INTERMED total score

The total score on the INTERMED is 34, which is in the high range and supports the argument made for coordination of care and a case manager (see also the later section in this article on scientific evaluation of the INTERMED).

Fig. 4 illustrates the visual representation of the risks.

The clinical data related to the scoring also can be organized in the following way; this method may be helpful, for example, when the patient

Subject: Glover
Admission/referral date: 2006-04-03 00:00
Docter/nurse: 1743
Department: Cardiology

Reason for referral/admission: Chestpain

score: 33	History		Current state		Prognoses	
Biological	Chronicity		Severity of symptoms		Complications and life-threat	
	Diagnostic dilemma		Diagnostic challenge			
Psychological	Restrictions in coping		Resistance to treatment		Restrictions in integration	
	Psychiatric dysfunction		Psychiatric symptoms			
Social	Restrictions in integration		Residential instability		Social vulnerability	
	Social dysfunctioning		Restrictions of network			
Health care	Intensity of treatment		Organisation of care		Coordination	
	Treatment experience		Appropriateness of referral			

☐ No vulnerability nor need to act

☐ Mild vulnerability and need for monitoring or prevention

▨ Moderate vulnerability and need for treatment or inclusion in treatment plan

■ Severe vulnerability and need for immediate action or intensive treatment

Fig. 4. Scoring of the case vignette of Mr. Glover.

should be referred to a different facility. In the electronic version, the previously described, computer-entered clinical information is organized automatically, as shown later (see also the later section in this article on "How to learn more about the INTERMED").

Biologic risks. Mr. Glover is a 55-year-old man who has been admitted through the emergency room to a cardiac ward for a myocardial infarction complicated by a ventricle tachycardia; the cardiac condition requires immobilization. Mr. Glover suffers from a chronic disease (hypertension), recently complicated by another chronic condition (heart disease resulting from a myocardial infarction). There have not been other episodes of physical illness in the last 5 years.

Social risks. Over the last 5 years, work has dominated his life to such extent that it has negatively influenced the relationship with his wife; they have lived separately for a month. The patient currently is living alone in a hotel room. Other than a sister and a colleague, he does not have people who will support him, nor does he have time for or interest in leisure activities.

Psychologic risks. From a psychologic perspective, Mr. Glover has denied his cardiac condition and tends to reduce tension with smoking and drinking. His history indicates an earlier episode of mood disorder and impaired coping after the separation from his first wife. Currently he presents substance-abuse problems concerning tobacco and alcohol and a depressive disorder. This psychologic state interferes with his compliance with medical treatment as reflected in the recent inability to take medication on a regular basis and his behavior, which represents a risk for his cardiac condition.

Health care risks. In the last 5 years Mr. Glover has been admitted for a first myocardial infarction and has been treated by a primary care physician and a cardiologist. At the moment he does not see any medical or other caretakers. His trust in doctors has been negatively influenced by two earlier incidents.

Prognoses. Biologic prognosis: the patient suffers from a chronic condition and in the future might experience permanent substantial limitations in activities of daily living.

Psychologic prognosis: the patient has a psychiatric disorder requiring psychiatric care; he suffers from depression, which is complicated by various other conditions, such as substance abuse, social isolation, and a serious medical illness.

Social prognosis: because of his current physical condition and the social situation, the patient has a serious risk of a temporary admission to a facility.

Health care: taking into account the risks factors in the various domains, the patient should be considered as complex, requiring different specialist consultations and care coordination, including mental health care.

Treatment plan. Biologic level: depending on the stabilization of the circulation in the first 24 hours, the patient's cardiac condition will be evaluated according to protocol. The cardiologist regards his postdischarge functional prognosis to be in the range of New York Heart Association classification 1 to 2. For the first 24 hours the patient should be monitored for physical symptoms of alcohol withdrawal by observing his sleeping patterns, although the risk seems relatively low. Given the overall situation, a low dosage of benzodiazepines will be prescribed for 3 to 5 days to prevent distress, which could influence his cardiac condition negatively. After stabilization, the patient should be referred to a cardiac rehabilitation program, followed by regular medical appointments.

Psychologic level: a psychiatric consultant should assess the patient and evaluate the interrelation between coping, compliance, substance abuse, and depression. As a result of this assessment it should be decided who should initiate treatment, at what time, and of what type. Because compliance with treatment is crucial in this patient, the primary focus of the intervention should be to motivate the patient to obtain psychologic treatment. Depending on the results of the contacts with the sister and his wife, the integration of these persons in the psychiatric treatment plan should be considered.

Social level: the patient's wife should be invited to explore further his social and relational situation. Based on the results of this exploration, the outcome of his physical condition, and the results of the psychiatric assessment, decisions on the location of postdischarge treatment should be made: psychiatric transfer, rehabilitation clinic, or ambulant treatment.

Health care level: a multidisciplinary case conference should be organized in the next days to integrate the results of the different consultants (rehabilitation, psychiatry, and social work); later an assigned case manager should coordinate the treatment program.

Fig. 5 shows a form for recording a treatment plan.

Scientific evaluation of the INTERMED

There are different approaches to developing and evaluating measurement instruments. The essence of classic test theory is that the measure of

Patient identification   **DIAGNOSTICS AND TREATMENT**

Date	:
MD	:
Nurse	:

	DIAGNOSTICS	☑	TREATMENT	☑
BIOLOGICAL	Cardiac monitoring		Cardiac protocol	
	Withdrawal monitoring		R/ Oxazepam 10-25 mgr ttd	
	Sleep monitoring		R/ Oxazepam 25-50 mgr AN	
			PM:	
			- R/ antidepressants	
			- Cardiac rehabilitation	
			☐ **RESTRICTIONS OF TREATMENT**	
PSYCHOLOGICAL	Monitor mood and suicidal thoughts		Motivational intervention to secure	
	Psychiatric assessment :		psychological Tx for coping,	
	- substance abuse, depression		compliance, substance abuse and	
	- compliance and coping		depression	
	Assessment of relation with wife		Consider participation of wife	
SOCIAL	Assessment of housing situation		Plan discharge management	
			based on findings of consultants	
	PARTICIPANTS		**Activities**	
HEALTH CARE	Psychiatrist		Case conference after initial consults	
	Rehab specialist		Assign casemanager	
	Social worker			

Fig. 5. Form for recording treatment plan.

any construct involves the use of all possible items that can be identified to measure the target construct accurately. Item-analysis evaluates the degree to which items in a given set correlate (a correlation between 0.30–0.60 is desirable: items measuring a similar construct without being redundant [35]). Factor analysis identifies the underlying structure of the relationship among sampled items and evaluates whether the items share a common construct. Testing of reliability and validity (especially construct validity based on statistical evidence) complements this evaluation (see article in this issue by Lyons). In contrast to classic test theory, items-response theory approaches the problem by evaluating whether the measurement has the ability to distinguish between different people reliably, all along a continuum; its goal is to identify a set of items that allows the precise measurement of an individual on the latent continuum or trait. From a pragmatic perspective, however, classic test theory and items-response theory value measures that have a large number of items and measure a single dimension, leading to longer and one-dimensional measures.

These two traditional approaches to developing and evaluating psychometric measurement instruments thus have common problems: (1) their usefulness in clinical practice is limited, because most clinical conditions and also outcomes have more than a single dimension; (2) there is little time and motivation to implement one-dimensional and long measures; (3) they are diagnostic instruments with limited relevance for decision making and treatment planning; and (4) they have been produced for research purposes and have not been developed under real-world conditions. For these reasons, one can easily imagine that the objectives of the INTERMED, a biopsychosocial assessment instrument for case complexity, which serves as a decision-support and treatment-planning tool, cannot be based solely on classic test theory and items-response analysis but must be complemented by the clinimetric and communimetric approaches.

Clinimetrics, in contrast to psychometrics, aims to convert "intangible clinical phenomena into formal specified measurement" [36]. For clinimetric measures, items are selected using clinical rather than statistical criteria, scoring is simple and readily interpretable, variables are heterogeneous, and face validity is required. The Global Assessment of Functioning Scale is an example [37]. Clinimetric instruments tend not to be very sensitive to change and usually are unable to embrace the complexity of a given clinical state. Communimetrics aims to integrate in a measure elements that facilitate easy and accurate communication of relevant results; this integration requires that communimetric measures have a high face validity, high interrater reliability, high concurrent and predictive validity, and results that can be used immediately for decision making, treatment planning, and outcome measurement. As described at the beginning of this article, the INTERMED approach shares the objectives of clinimetrics and communimetrics, but its development and scientific evaluation also draw on classic test theory relevant for psychometric measurements. In the following discussion, the scientific aspects of the INTERMED are summarized; for a detailed description, the reader is referred to the existing literature referenced in the text.

Initially, an item pool characterizing biopsychosocial case complexity was selected on the basis of face validity and evidence from the literature that a given item is known to increase case complexity and associated health care use. As an example, the item "Chronicity" (history, biologic domain) has been selected, because the distinction between acute and chronic diseases has proven helpful for the conceptualization of somatic diseases and the patient's care needs, especially in the elderly. The approach to treating chronic illnesses cannot be treated based solely on standardized, scientific evidence. An evidence-based approach must be complemented by an adjustment of treatment goals that are realistic for a given individual. Management of diabetes in an elderly man who suffered from the consequences of the Second World War in his youth and who is slightly depressed after the death of his wife cannot follow the same lines as the management of a diabetic young school teacher who engages in sports activities on a regular basis. In addition, chronic diseases, in contrast to episodes of acute illness, increase the risk of a comorbid psychiatric disturbance, because the prevalence of psychiatric disturbances is increased in chronic medical illnesses. Thus "Chronicity" has been selected for the INTERMED item pool, because it reflects an important variable when describing biopsychosocial case complexity.

Subsequently the INTERMED item pool was reduced and validated by means of correlations with existing longer, one-dimensional instruments [35,38]. Because no reference standard for the assessment of case complexity existed, in the evaluation of the concurrent validity the authors compared the INTERMED with a variety of other instruments that were valid for some of the dimensions of the INTERMED, such as the Short Form-36 (SF-36) Physical Health Component Score in the biologic domain, the SF-36 Mental Health Component Score and the Hospital Anxiety and Depression Scale in the psychologic domain, and scales measuring characteristics such as social support and social isolation in the social domain [14,39]. This approach was based on a psychometric evaluation of concurrent validity. In contrast with a purely clinimetric approach, items reflecting subjective data were not excluded, because complaints perceived and expressed by the patient are relevant for the assessment of case complexity and especially for health care use. The first steps of the INTERMED development thus followed combined psychometric and clinimetric approach, favoring the selection of clinically meaningful and face-valid items that can be used easily in clinical practice.

With regard to reliability, the evaluation of the INTERMED again followed psychometric approaches by testing internal consistency and interrater and test–retest reliability [38]. After the first interrater reliability study with the INTERMED [14], a final version was developed, which then was tested in a sample of patients who had varying somatic illnesses. Patients were double-scored by two raters, a psychologist and a psychiatric nurse, based on a review of the medical chart and a patient interview conducted by one in the presence of the other. The two raters showed high agreement, as indicated by a κ of 0.85 [40]. Temporal stability of the INTERMED was assessed in outpatients who had multiple sclerosis, with an interval of 1 year between the two assessments and without a specific intervention other than care as usual [41]. The correlation between the two assessments was moderate to good (indicated by a κ of 0.60) reflecting the fact that the INTERMED is a rather stable measure.

As in classic test theory, data from several of the INTERMED studies in different somatic patient populations were pooled to evaluate internal consistency [42]. In the total sample (N = 1104), Cronbach's α was 0.87 (95% confidence interval, 0.86–0.89); for the individual samples, α ranged from 0.78 to 0.94. The findings gave sufficient support for the reliability of the INTERMED and the adequacy of the total score to describe biopsychosocial case complexity.

Predictive validity, as required for an instrument that should provide clinically meaningful information (clinimetric approach), was studied by selecting relevant outcome variables in several specific patient populations (for a summary, see Table 2). In patients admitted to a general medical ward, those classified by the INTERMED as having a high degree of case complexity were found to have a doubled length of hospital stay and increased use of medications, nurse interventions, and specialist consultations [43]. The findings were replicated later [44]; in addition, poorer quality of life at discharge was documented for the complex patients. In patients who had diabetes, INTERMED scores correlated with HbA1c values assessed 6 months before and 3 and 9 months after the INTERMED interview [45]. In a sample of patients who had low back pain who had participated in a 3-week functional rehabilitation program or who had applied for disability compensation, INTERMED scores were significantly higher in those applying for disability compensation [14]. In patients receiving dialysis INTERMED scores were associated with low quality of life at 1-year follow-up [39] that was unrelated to severity of illness at baseline. In outpatients who had multiple sclerosis, INTERMED scores were associated with measures of disability and with the number of disciplines proposed in the multidisciplinary treatment plan [46]. In patients suffering from rheumatoid arthritis, INTERMED scores, in contrast to other measures evaluating severity of illness, predicted health care use upon follow-up [47]. These data confirmed the ability of the INTERMED to detect complex patients at risk for decreased treatment response and increased health care use.

Overview of INTERMED studies

As a criterion for the detection of complex cases in general medical wards, a cut-off point of 20/21 was identified [44], based on an optimized prediction of patients with poor outcomes at discharge from the hospital.

Table 2
Overview of INTERMED validation studies

	N	Definition of Poor Outcome	Area Under the Curve	P-value	Prevalence of Poor Outcome (%)	Sensitivity	Specificity	Odds ratio[f]	95% Confidence Interval	P-value
Internal medicine	152	SF-36 < 50[a]	0.69	<.0001	51	0.58	0.76	4.45	2.22–8.94	<.0001
Multiple sclerosis	72	EDSS[g] > 4[b]	0.75	<.0001	53	0.65	0.94	8.89	1.85–42.63	<.0001
Dialysis	46	SF-36 < 50[c]	0.76	.002	50	0.61	0.74	4.41	1.26–15.41	.02
Low back pain	102	Applying for disability compensation[d]	0.89	<.0001	50	0.94	0.45	13.14	3.62–47.76	<.01
Diabetes mellitus	55	HbA1c > 8.3[e]	0.65	.06	51	0.71	0.52	2.32	0.76–7.08	.14

Abbreviation: SF-36, Short-Form 36.
[a] Assessed at discharge (INTERMED at admission).
[b] Cross-sectional design.
[c] Assessed at 1-year follow-up.
[d] Cross-sectional design.
[e] Mean HbA1c over 3, 6, and 9 months follow-up.
[f] Odds for a poor outcome for patients with INTERMED score beyond cut-off criterion (20/21).
[g] Expanded Disability Status Scale.
Data from de Jonge P, Huyse FJ, Slaets JP, et al. Operationalization of biopsychosocial case complexity in general health care: the INTERMED project. Aust N Z J Psychiatry 2005;39(9):797.

The identification of a cut-off point is contrary to the statement that the instrument to assess case complexity should result in a continuous score. In addition, any cut-off point of a continuous score is arbitrary, to a certain extent, can result in bias [48], and—with regard to the INTERMED—should depend on the specific case mix of the sample and the resources available to deal with complex patients. Therefore, if INTERMED cut-off scores have to be used in a specific clinical practice, the authors recommend using a cut-off score based on empiric grounds.

This article has presented the main psychometric and clinimetric properties of the INTERMED, but the communimetric elements have been discussed only in part. The previously mentioned communimetric characteristics of the INTERMED are its face validity, interrater reliability, and concurrent and predictive validity. The communimetric properties of the INTERMED also concern its relevance for patients, who expressed their satisfaction with the interview (authors' unpublished data) and the simple manual containing the described anchor points that can help clinicians find a common language when using the INTERMED in daily clinical practice and multidisciplinary case conferences. In addition, the communimetric characteristics of the INTERMED also have been demonstrated by the feasibility of conducting a multicenter study involving different European countries [49]. Finally, the communimetric elements of the INTERMED concern the objective that its results can be used directly for decision making and treatment planning. While randomized clinical trials currently are being conducted to evaluate the INTERMED as a decision-support and treatment-planning tool [50], the INTERMED is being implemented in two different clinical settings, in a university clinic (the internal medicine ward of the University Medical Center Groningen and a neurologic ward in the Vrije Universiteit Medical Center in Amsterdam, both in the Netherlands) and in a regional rehabilitation clinic (the National Insurance of Traffic Accidents [SUVA] rehabilitation clinic in Sion, Switzerland) (Luthi F, Deriaz O, Stiefel F, et al. Biopsychosocial "case complexity" and treatment outcome after musculoskeletal injuries: a prospective study utilizing the INTERMED; unpublished article).

The crucial question whether implementation of the INTERMED leads to improved outcomes for the complex medically ill has been addressed in two earlier studies. In the first study, the authors investigated the effects of implementing psychiatric interventions on a general medical admission ward by means of a stepped detection-and-treatment strategy conducted by a consultation-liaison nurse in terms of reducing length of hospital stay and improving quality of life at discharge, as compared with usual care. A significant effect of the intervention on quality of life was found, and in patients age 65 years or older a reduction in median length of hospital stay from 16 to 11.5 days was established. These data suggest that screening for risk of increased health care might improve outcomes in general medical inpatients. Because of the design of the study, which includes an historic control group, these findings should be considered preliminary and confirmed in a larger, multicenter, randomized controlled trial [51]. In a second study, patients discharged home after hospitalization in the general hospital were randomly assigned to usual care or to a nurse-led home-based case management intervention, based on a health needs assessment with the INTERMED. No significant differences were found in rehospitalization, care use, quality of life, and psychologic functioning after 24 weeks of follow-up. The primary reason for the lack of effectiveness in this trial is that the case manager implemented the intervention in relative isolation, which hampered its effectiveness, instead of being fully integrated with the existing health care delivery (Latour CHM, de Vos R, Huyse FJ, De et al. Effectiveness of postdischarge case management in general medical outpatients; randomized controlled trial; unpublished article).

Recently the limitations of these studies have been addressed in a firm, randomized, controlled trial involving inpatients admitted to a rheumatology ward and diabetic outpatients. The hypothesis was that an early multidisciplinary intervention targeted at complex patients identified by and based on the INTERMED is superior to care as usual. Outcomes were related to subjective measures (quality of life), treatment response, and cost effectiveness. The results are being prepared for publication. Benefits have been observed with regard to the different outcomes mentioned [49]. Comparative epidemiologic studies evaluating health care benefits of implementing the INTERMED will complement the randomized clinical trials conducted up to now (Latour CHM, de Vos R, Huyse FJ, et al. Effectiveness of postdischarge case management in general medical outpatients; randomized controlled trial; unpublished article and [52]).

In addition to the scientific evaluation of the INTERMED mentioned previously, the instrument can be used in research protocols (eg, to control for case mix or for stratification of populations with differing degrees of case complexity) (see Box 1). Integration of the INTERMED in scientific projects could be of great help in interpreting outcome and identifying patients who would benefit most from a given intervention.

How to learn more about the INTERMED

The manual containing the clinical anchor points is now available in English, French, German, Dutch, Italian, Spanish, and Turkish. The English, French, German, and Dutch versions were developed in close collaboration with the founders of the INTERMED project. Subsequently, the Italian, Spanish, and Turkish versions were developed according to the professional standard of forward and blind backward translations. These manuals can be printed from the following website: www.INTERMEDfoundation.org. Japanese, Swedish and Hungarian versions are in process of validation.

In 2007 multilanguage web-based clinical and training facilities will become available to support clinical practice and multicenter research. This

---

Box 1. Research applications of the INTERMED

- Inclusion and exclusion criterion for intervention studies, using either the total score (cut-off) or combinations of variable scores
- Stratification
- Prediction of outcomes measures such as mortality, morbidity, quality of life
- Reduction of unexplained variance in randomized clinical trials (case-mix measure) leading to an increase of the power of the study and a smaller sample required to reach significance
- Control for possible confounders in randomized clinical trials leading to a better estimation of the effect-size
- A standardized procedure to design an individualized patient-oriented intervention, such as in case management studies

---

Information Technology (IT) application includes a medical problem list and the option of entering the clinical data collected during the interview in addition to the scoring, as well as the option of detailing the treatment plan. Related to these data-entry capabilities are report functions, including a function in which the information is presented in the format used for the case vignette of Mr. Glover and the cases given in Appendix 3.

Implementation of the INTERMED in clinical practice

As argued in the article by Huyse and colleagues in this issue, the primary step toward integrated medicine is the awareness by a medical/nursing team that integrated medicine benefits the complex patient. Implementation of the INTERMED method is similar to the initiation of a quality-management procedure. Presenting the details of quality management exceeds the scope of this article. Most important, implementation of the INTERMED in clinical practice is based on teamwork and requires an assigned group to guide and evaluate this process. As the team changes its approach from a classic disease-oriented focus to an integrated approach, the specific specialties of team members must be adjusted to the needs of the patients; for example, a mental health specialist should be an integral member of the team. In hospitals, contracts can be made between different services and departments (eg, in primary care arrangements need to be made with mental health organizations). Different types of such arrangements are described in the article in this issue by Wulsin and colleagues. Because the interventions of integrated care teams should be targeted, the indications for assessment and interventions described in this issue by Huyse and colleagues should be respected.

As a first step, a team could conduct a cohort study to identify the proportion of complex patients, their specific needs, and possible indicators for identification and subsequently decide upon specific competences to include in the team. The next question is who should be responsible for assessment. In inpatients, primary care, and outpatient clinics, trained nurses may be best suited conduct such assessments, in collaboration with physicians. In some settings, however—depending on local and cultural circumstances—physicians may conduct INTERMED interviews. The most important aspect of the implementation of the INTERMED method is interdisciplinary collaboration; visions from different professional perspectives must meet, and interdisciplinary communication should be enhanced. The "chasms" as described in the Institute of Medicine report [33] need to be counteracted by communication between departments or institutes and by interdisciplinary communication within a team. Therefore the integration of the collected information and its analyses in the admission/referral process is crucial for it to become the driving force guiding the therapeutic process. Multidisciplinary meetings will become part of the health service structure, and care consequently will shift from a professional to a patient perspective.

The clinical implementation of the INTERMED method began in 2003. It is currently implemented in several settings, and a variety of teams in several countries are working on implementing it. The INTERMED was first implemented in the admission department of general internal medicine of the University Medical Center in Groningen, The Netherlands. All patients admitted to this ward are screened with the INTERMED and are discussed in daily multidisciplinary rounds. During these rounds an outline of the treatment plan based on the results of the INTERMED is designed, including decisions on discharge within 48 hours or a longer admission with related transfer to a specialized ward. Transfers are accompanied by the INTERMED treatment plan. Because the INTERMED method is part of the clinical management system, all data are accessible at any time. Consultants such as psychiatrists, geriatricians, and social workers add pertinent information to the electronic INTERMED module to assure completeness of information. Reports can be printed for the transfer of individual patients or to provide an overview. In the University Medical Center in Groningen the implementation as part of a preassessment clinic for elective surgery is currently considered as a means to decrease perioperative complications. A similar procedure is followed on the neurologic department of the Vrije Universiteit medical center in Amsterdam. In contrast to its use in the department of internal medicine in Groningen, in Amsterdam the INTERMED method drives a weekly multidisciplinary meeting. Only patients who have a score above a cut-off point of 20/21 are discussed in this meeting. This procedure has reduced the duration of the meeting from 90 minutes to 45 minutes. On both the internal and the neurologic ward, INTERMED data collection became an integral part of the nurse chart [34]. The INTERMED is used in the Clinic of the National Insurance of Traffic Accidents (Sion,

Switzerland) for admission screening and related ongoing research [50]; the responsible physicians report that the implementation of the INTERMED has changed their practice, enhanced interdisciplinary communication, speeded up specialist consultations, and improved staff satisfaction. A primary care (home practitioner or general practitioner) project has been initiated in a lower socioeconomic area that has a high percentage of uninsured persons in the city of Utrecht, the Netherlands; the aim is to obtain a better idea of their specific treatment needs. A European multicenter outcome-prediction study in transplant patients is currently being conducted; its aim is to evaluate the benefits of implementing the INTERMED in this complex field. In the United States interest for the INTERMED has been expressed in the fields of health plans, pharmacy monitoring, and primary care.

Future development

The INTERMED method provides a conceptual framework and a basis for operationalizing effective and integrated multidisciplinary treatment targeted at the complex medically ill. As such it is relevant for health care providers, policy makers, hospital managers, and insurance companies and is most important for complex patients who have psychosocial comorbidities leading to diminished response to medical treatments. The first results of ongoing randomized trials confirm the benefits of implementing the INTERMED and driving a multidisciplinary treatment plan based on its results. Many steps still are needed to make the INTERMED method more accessible and to increase its implementation. For example, Web-based training based on INTERMED interviews of simulated patients should help future users to learn how to use the method. It is hoped that the INTERMED project will contribute to a paradigm shift from a specialty-oriented to a patient-centered model of interdisciplinary care, foster comprehensive assessment and treatment of the complex medically ill, and thereby contribute to fulfilling the six aims and 10 new rules formulated by the Institute of Medicine for the future of integrated care for the complex medically ill (see the Preface of this issue and [33]).

Appendix 1

INTERMED variables and their clinical anchor points

The INTERMED assesses complexity. Complexity is defined the presence of coexisting conditions (biologic, psychologic, social, or related to the health care system) that interfere with standard care and require a shift from standard care to individualized care. Whenever a variable is rated, in addition to the clinical anchor points as defined below, one should ask, "Will this information result in interferences with the standard care?"

All variables in the history concern a timeframe of the last 5 years. There is one exception: the variable psychiatric dysfunctioning covers a lifetime perspective.

Biologic history

Chronicity
>   0 Less than 3 months of physical dysfunctioning
>   1 More than 3 months of physical dysfunctioning or several periods of less than 3 months
>   2 A chronic disease
>   3 Several chronic diseases

Diagnostic dilemma
>   0 No periods of diagnostic complexity
>   1 Diagnoses and the etiology were clarified quickly
>   2 Diagnostic dilemma was solved, but only with considerable diagnostic effort
>   3 Diagnostic dilemma not solved despite considerable diagnostic efforts

Current biologic state

Severity of symptoms
>   0 No symptoms, or symptoms reversible without intensive medical efforts
>   1 Mild but notable symptoms that do not interfere with current functioning
>   2 Moderate to severe symptoms that interfere with current functioning
>   3 Severe symptoms leading to inability to perform any functional activities

Diagnostic challenge
>   0 Clear diagnosis
>   1 Clear differential diagnosis
>   2 Complex differential diagnosis in which a diagnosis from a biologic perspective is to be expected
>   3 Complex differential diagnosis in which no diagnosis is to be expected from a biologic perspective

Psychologic history

Restrictions in coping
>   0 No restrictions in coping: ability to manage stress adequately, no impairment of medical treatment
>   1 Mild restrictions in coping that cause mild to moderate distress in patient and/or relatives or health care providers (eg, complaining behavior)

2 Moderate restrictions in coping that cause severe emotional distress in patients and/or relatives or health care providers (eg, aggressive behavior or substance abuse without negative biopsychosocial effects) and/or impairment of medical treatment (eg, prolonged denial)

3 Severe limitations in coping that produce serious psychiatric symptomatology (eg, substance abuse with negative biopsychosocial effects, self-mutilation, or attempted suicide) and impairment of medical treatment

Psychiatric dysfunction

0 No psychiatric dysfunction
1 Psychiatric dysfunction without clear effects on daily functioning
2 Psychiatric dysfunction with clear effects on daily functioning
3 Psychiatric admissions and/or permanent effects on daily functioning

Current psychologic state

Resistance to treatment

0 Interested in receiving treatment and willing to cooperate actively
1 Some ambivalence although willing to cooperate with treatment
2 Considerable resistance (eg, noncompliance, hostility, or indifference towards health care professionals)
3 Active resistance against medical care

Psychiatric symptoms

0. No psychiatric symptoms
1. Mild psychiatric symptoms (eg, problems in concentrating or feeling tense)
2. Psychiatric symptoms (eg, anxiety, depression, or confusion)
3. Psychiatric symptoms with behavioral disturbances (eg, violence or self-injurious behavior)

Social history

Restrictions in integration

0 Employed (including housekeeping, retirement, studying) and has leisure activities
1 Employed (including housekeeping, retirement, studying) without leisure activities
2 At least 6 months unemployed, with leisure activities
3 At least 6 months unemployed, without leisure activities

Social dysfunctioning

0 No social disruption
1 Mild social dysfunctioning; interpersonal problems
2 Moderate social dysfunctioning (eg, unable to initiate or maintain social relations)

3 Severe social dysfunctioning (eg, involvement in disruptive social relations or social isolation)

Current social state

Residential instability
0 Stable housing situation; fully capable of independent living
1 Stable housing situation with support of others (eg, an institutional setting or home care)
2 Unstable housing situation; change of current living situation is required
3 Unstable housing situation; immediate change is necessary

Restrictions of network
Persons on sickness leave are scored as working. Those receiving disability compensation are scored as not working. Students and persons engaged in unpaid labor are scored as working.

0 Good contacts with family, work and friends
1 Restrictions in one of the domains
2 Restrictions in two of the domains
3 Restrictions in three of the domains

History of health care

Intensity of treatment
0 Fewer than four contacts with physicians per year
1 Four or more contacts with physicians or one specialist per year
2 Different specialists or a hospital admission
3 Several hospitalizations or stay on ICU, complex surgery, or stay on rehabilitation unit

Treatment experience
0 No problems with health care professionals
1 Negative experience with health care providers (self or relatives)
2 Requests for second opinions or changing contacts with doctors
3 Repeated conflicts with doctors, or involuntary admissions

Current state of health care

Organization of care
0 One specialist (general health care or mental health care)
1 Different specialists in the general health care system
2 Both general and mental health specialists
3 Transfer from another hospital

Appropriateness of referral
0 Regular referral or planned admission
1 Unplanned referral or emergency admission

2 Able to plan a strategy for treatment but not capable of providing optimal care

3 Unable to plan a strategy for treatment

Prognoses

Complications and threats to life

0 No limitations in activities of daily living

1 Mild limitations in activities of daily living

2 Chronic condition and/or permanent substantial limitations in activities of daily living

3 Severe physical complications and functional deficits, serious risk of death

Mental health threat

0 No psychiatric disorder

1 Mild psychiatric disorder (eg, such as adjustment disorder, anxiety, feeling blue, substance abuse, or cognitive disturbance)

2 Moderate psychiatric disorder requiring psychiatric care

3 Severe psychiatric disorder requiring psychiatric admission

Social vulnerability

0 No changes in the living situation; no additional care needs

1 No changes in the living situation but additional home (nursing) care or social work assistance needed

2 Temporary admission to facility/institution

3 Permanent admission to facility/institution

Coordination of health care

The organization of the present health care system is taken into account in rating this item

0 No problems in the organization of care

1 Minor efforts needed to organize care: multidisciplinary care that is easy to organize

2 Moderate efforts to organize care: multidisciplinary care that is difficult to organize

3 Severe efforts needed to organize care: need for case conference and/or coordination of care

Appendix 2

Leading questions for the INTERMED interview (examples)

Now, first of all, I would like to better understand how you feel physically?

I will tell you what I know about the reason for your admission and your current state. You should correct me when I am wrong.

Now I would like to know how you felt emotionally during the last week.

I would like to have some more information concerning physical illnesses and treatments in the past 5 years.

Who are the doctors who have been taking care for you in the last 5 years?

Have you ever seen a psychiatrist or have there been periods in your life that you have been anxious, depressed, or confused?

Now who are the doctors, nurses, social workers, or psychologists whom you are currently seeing and who take care for you?

Have there been issues with doctors during the last 5 years that gave you a bad feeling to such an extent that it might interfere with your trust in doctors?

I would like to know how you follow your doctor's recommendations. Are you a person who, generally speaking, is inclined to do what doctors say?

Now I would like to change the subject and ask you how you currently live.

Now I would like to know what kind of person you are. Generally speaking, are you an easygoing person?

Now, coming to the end of the interview, I would like to ask you about your smoking and drinking habits and their relation to the current problems.

Do you think we missed any pertinent information?

Finally. I would like to know how you have experienced this interview. Do you think that this will be helpful information, or did you think this was inappropriate?

Appendix 3

Case examples and scoring sheets

Three cases are presented to illustrate the rationale of using the INTERMED in clinical practice. After a short description of the information available at referral or admission and the information obtained from the patient, the scoring of the INTERMED is provided. The readers are referred to the description of the clinical anchor points in Appendix 1 and are invited to perform the scoring and check their results using the proposed scoring presented at the end of this Appendix. Finally, for each case a summarized case vignette, as used for multidisciplinary case conferences, referral, or discharge letters, is provided, followed by a proposal for a treatment plan.

OPERATIONALIZING INTEGRATED CARE

Patient 1: admission for diarrhea and some other complications

Reason for admission

The patient, a 27-year-old woman, was admitted to the department of gastroenterology for the evaluation of diarrhea. There are several reasons for the admission. First, in the last month extensive diagnostic evaluations have been made, but a final diagnosis is still to be determined. Second, the patient's condition has declined, and she has lost about 10 kg in the last month. Third, the patient has informed her doctor that she is almost incapable of doing anything at home. She has suffered from systemic lupus erythematosus (SLE) for about 4 years and is being treated by a nephrologist, because her kidneys were the primary location of the disease. There is a gradual decline of the kidney function. A relationship between the diarrhea and the SLE is expected but has not yet been confirmed.

Additional information

During the admission the following information is obtained. Although the patient is silent during the admission process, she starts to cry when the nurse suggests that she must have been in an awful situation, being so ill at home. She replies, "How would you feel? I have been ill ever since I was married!" She then tells the nurse that in the beginning the complaints were vague. One doctor had suggested the stress of the marriage as a cause. Later, another doctor suggested the possibility of chronic fatigue. She then visited a neurologist, because a friend suggested that she might suffer from multiple sclerosis. The neurologist, after carefully listening and reviewing the earlier reports, referred her to an internist, suggesting a rheumatic disease. At first the internists, although they found abnormalities in her blood, could not find a diagnosis. Finally the diagnosis of systemic lupus erythematosus was made, and treatment with corticosteroids and another drug was started, because her kidneys did not function well. Although the doctors were satisfied with the results, and she felt a little better, she hated the bloated look induced by the medication. Therefore, in the beginning, she stopped her medication a few times; now she still has resistance and doubts but basically complies with what doctors prescribe.

In the course of their marriage it also became clear that she was not able to get pregnant. She therefore visited an infertility clinic about 2 years ago. After all kinds of investigations the doctors concluded that, because of her illness, she could not be admitted to a fertilization program; her chances of becoming pregnant were regarded as minimal. Although she asked the doctors to discuss this issue with her nephrologist, no action was taken, and she was afraid of being perceived as difficult and did not ask again. As a consequence of the diagnostic confusion in the past she does not really trust doctors, although she trusts her nephrologist and is inclined to follow his advice.

From being a cheerful adolescent she gradually became a person who had a negative self image: that she was not a good partner for her husband, could not have children, and was always tired. The information received about 2 years ago that she was not able to bear a child induced very negative feelings, and she attempted suicide using her husband's painkillers. She was unsuccessful, and she did not inform anyone of this attempt.

The relation with her husband deteriorated during the last 5 years, because he could not accept the idea of not having children. Consequently they often had quarrels and even fights. He even hit her a few times. The family did not understand her staying with her husband and turned away. The couple has almost no friends. The patient did not have many interests but succeeded getting a volunteer job preparing drinks in a daycare center for children. For last month she has not been able to perform at all. The diarrhea made her feel weak. Her mood declined; her thoughts were focused on the course her life had taken, and she often thought, "Why do I take all this medication?" Often she thought she would be better off dead.

Scoring case 1

The reader is invited to score this case using scoring sheet provided in Fig. 6 and the clinical anchor points described in Appendix 1 and to check the results as presented at the end of Appendix 3.

Case vignette

The patient is a 27-year-old woman who was admitted to the department of gastroenterology for diarrhea, because this condition represents a diagnostic problem and because the patient feels weak and is not able to care for herself. Several years ago, she was diagnosed as having SLE with a kidney location, but several referrals and quite some time were required to obtain the diagnosis. Patient is living in her own apartment with her husband. Their relation is complicated, because she is always ill and is not able to have children. Her condition has resulted in quarrels and fights. They almost divorced. Because of her illness, the patient has never been able to work, but she did perform some volunteer work. There are almost no social contacts. She has negative feelings about herself. Sometime ago, when she realized she

	P	C	P
B	0 1 2 3 0 1 2 3	0 1 2 3 0 1 2 3	0 1 2 3
P	0 1 2 3 0 1 2 3	0 1 2 3 0 1 2 3	0 1 2 3
S	0 1 2 3 0 1 2 3	0 1 2 3 0 1 2 3	0 1 2 3
HC	0 1 2 3 0 1 2 3	0 1 2 3 0 1 2 3	0 1 2 3

Fig. 6. Scoring sheet for Case 1.

would never be able to have children, she tried to commit suicide using medication. During recent years she had felt a little blue most of the time. Currently, she admits to feeling depressed and to thoughts that she would better be dead. A nephrologist, a gastroenterologist, and a gynecologist have treated the patient. The first two are her current caretakers. The patient's respect for doctors suffered when several doctors involved in the assessment of her complaints provided different but seemingly inappropriate answers. She trusts her current physicians, but her general trust in doctors and what they can do is diminished. Basically, the patient is compliant, although there is some resistance because of the side effects of the medication and the deterioration of her situation.

Treatment plan
Biologic. This patient suffers from a complex medical illness complicated by new symptoms of previously unclear origin. The available diagnostic procedures should be re-evaluated. Because diarrhea might also be a symptom of a psychiatric disorder (anxiety and depression), this could be an alternative explanation. Because the patient is weak and has suffered weight loss, a dietician and a physiotherapist should be consulted.

Psychologic. The patient is psychologically vulnerable. Most probably she suffers from a depressive disorder, which should be confirmed by a psychiatric consultation. This consultation is specifically necessary, because she has a history with a suicide attempt. The loss of vitality may be caused by the physical illness, the infertility, depression, a bad relationship with her partner, and withdrawal from family members. Another contributing etiologic factor might be the medication used for the SLE. A specific focus therefore should be treatment of the depression and assurance of compliance. Psychiatric medication should be adjusted to her physical illness. Tricyclic antidepressants might have an advantage over selective serotonin reuptake inhibitors because of their specific effects on the gut function. Furthermore the ward staff should be instructed in how to approach the patient, including her physical activity training. In addition involvement of the partner in the psychologic treatment of the patient should be considered.

Social. As part of the psychiatric assessment and treatment, interventions should be considered to counteract her social vulnerability. Depending on the outcome of the physical evaluation, the effects of the initiated treatment, and the results of the psychiatric assessment, a postdischarge plan should be made.

Organization of care. As indicated by the high total score (35), this case is highly complex with interactions between severe physical and psychiatric illness. Coordination between the different providers of care is required. A multidisciplinary case conference is necessary as soon as the results of the psychiatric, dietarian, and physiotherapy consultations are available. During the patient's hospital stay, a coordinator of care should be considered. When the patient is discharged to her home, postdischarge coordination of care is required.

Patient 2: evaluation of drain for normal-pressure hydrocephalus

Reason for admission

The patient is a 72-year-old man. He is admitted to the hospital for the evaluation of his ventriculo-peritoneal drain on request of the general practitioner after telephone consultation with the patient's neurosurgeon. The neurosurgeon evaluated the patient in the emergency room and decided there that an admission is necessary because there are clear signs of drain dysfunction. Patient was admitted 2 years ago for the placement of a drain for a normal-pressure hydrocephalus (NPH). The etiology of the NPH is most probably traumatic. A year before the patient had a bicycle accident in which he fractured a leg and had a cerebral contusion.

Additional information

At the end of the first day of admission the neurosurgeon and the nurse who admitted the patient collected the following information from the patient's wife. Before the operation he always had good physical health and has almost never seen a doctor. He had worked as the chief of financial administration in a firm with 100 employees. He had not been an easygoing man, because he was rather strict and stubborn, which resulted in conflicts and job changes. Retirement had been difficult for him because he missed his work. Through a neighbor he became a member of a bridge club. It was there that he had started to drink. The amount of his drinking had made his wife and also members of the club somewhat concerned. His accident occurred after one of the nights at the club.

After his hospitalization it had taken intensive work by his wife to get him in good shape again. Over the course of a year after coming home, he gradually developed walking difficulties, urinary incontinence, and memory problems. In addition the patient became easily irritated and difficult for his wife to manage. The general practitioner who was consulted suggested that the problems were all related to alcohol and advised the patient to stop his alcohol intake. Because the same general practitioner had missed the diagnosis of rheumatoid arthritis in the patient's wife, saying that her complaints were stress related, the wife had been dissatisfied with his suggestion and consulted another general practitioner with the patient. This general practitioner referred the patient to a neurologist to evaluate the effects of the cranial trauma.

The neurologist diagnosed an NPH and referred the patient to the neurosurgeon, who confirmed the NPH and recommended surgery. The admission for the surgery was associated with problems. The patient had been confused after being admitted and after the operation. There were signs of a delirium with as etiologic factors the operation, but alcohol withdrawal probably was involved as well. After about 2 weeks both physical and psychologic functions improved, and the patient was discharged to his home. The alcohol abuse had not been addressed further.

The last visit to the neurosurgeon had been about 6 months ago. During that visit the patient had to wait about an hour and concluded that this was his last visit, because he perceived the surgeon as passive and not doing much too help him. He had also stopped his visits to the club. The couple does not have offspring. There is telephone contact with family members at anniversaries.

The current period of deterioration started about 2 weeks ago. His wife informed the general practitioner that there were again signs comparable with the period before the NPH operation: walking became more difficult, and the patient became incontinent again. In addition, the patient, who was always difficult and quickly irritated, became even more difficult. He had threatened his wife about involving doctors and was increasingly drinking more. In the last few days he seemed to display a general sense of confusion, stopped drinking, could not remember what happened during the day, and was disoriented in time. He had been too ill to actively resist the ambulance personnel who came to bring him to the hospital. His wife informed the neurosurgeon that, whatever his findings and the results of surgery were, she would not be inclined to have him as a patient at home because she was afraid of him and unable to handle him, particularly because her rheumatoid arthritis had deteriorated. During the first day of admission the patient became irritated and threatened the nurses. He demanded to be released, saying he would otherwise summon the police. It was evident that he was disoriented in time and place and did not quite understand what was going on. Antipsychotic medication had been necessary to restrain him.

Scoring case 2

The reader is invited to score this case using the scoring sheet provided in Fig. 7 and clinical anchor points described in Appendix 1 and to check the results as presented at the end of Appendix 3.

Case vignette

The patient is a 72-year-old man admitted through an emergency procedure to the department of neurosurgery for the evaluation of the functioning of a drain for an earlier diagnosed and operated NPH. The reasons for doubts about its function were recent behavioral changes. The surgeon is quite confident about the diagnosis. Except for the NPH, which is trauma related, patient does not suffer from other physical diseases. The initial diagnosis of NPH was somewhat delayed. The patient is living with his wife, but she is unable to manage him in his current state and refuses to have him back at home. The couple does not have children, and their social contacts have diminished in the last years. Before retirement the patient was

	P	C	P
B	0 1 2 3 0 1 2 3	0 1 2 3 0 1 2 3	0 1 2 3
P	0 1 2 3 0 1 2 3	0 1 2 3 0 1 2 3	0 1 2 3
S	0 1 2 3 0 1 2 3	0 1 2 3 0 1 2 3	0 1 2 3
HC	0 1 2 3 0 1 2 3	0 1 2 3 0 1 2 3	0 1 2 3

Fig. 7. Scoring sheet for Case 2.

a financial administrator and later had some contacts in the bridge club. Because he was not an easygoing man, there were often conflicts at home. He was quickly irritated and started to drink increasingly at the bridge club. The patient experienced delirium during his earlier admission. In the days before and at this admission, the patient was confused and agitated. During the last years, the patient had some difficult contacts with health care providers. He had been admitted for the surgery but later stopped the contacts with the neurosurgeon. Currently only his general practitioner sees him. The patient's trust in doctors is reduced because of the course of the diagnostic process for the NPH, and his compliance with medical recommendations is impaired.

Treatment plan
Biologic. The patient suffers from a chronic physical condition that might be complicated by serious physical impairment. His current condition requires treatment of alcohol withdrawal, an evaluation of the function of the drain, and probably an operation. The course of the physical illness will have direct consequences for the current and long-term psychologic functioning of the patient.

Psychologic. The patient has indications of a serious psychiatric disturbance, including behavioral risks, with indications for immediate treatment. The patient is at risk of having or developing delirium caused by the NPH and alcohol abuse/withdrawal. Moreover there may be chronic cognitive impairment compatible with the development of a dementia. Because the patient is confused, he is not able to comply; this inability should be addressed actively to avoid further deterioration. Consequently the compliance should be enhanced by external factors, such as a stringent and probably parenteral medication regime. In addition, the prevention of injury and the instruction of family and staff about how to approach the patient according to the principles of delirium management is necessary. Interventions to prevent further psychologic deterioration during hospitalization are required. A long-term strategy is indicated to monitor and eventually ameliorate the cognitive capacity and the consequences of his character change.

Social. Rehabilitation through a nursing home should be considered, but placement in a nursing home might be the final outcome. Therefore additional information on the patient's housing situation and his wife's functional capacity is needed.

Organization of care. Because there is a combination of disturbances (high INTERMED score: 35) that interact with each other, and because of the patient's age, health care should provided by a multidisciplinary team including, in addition to the basic neurosurgery team, a geriatrician or a psychiatrist, depending on local policy, and a social worker. After emergency treatment for the withdrawal and the delirium, a case conference should be organized to plan long-term care and to assign a case manager. This planning is dependent upon the outcome of the neurosurgical/geriatric/psychiatric assessment and the information collected by the social worker. Preferably the care coordinator should be a geriatric nurse.

Patient 3: headache after an accident

Reason for visit

The patient is a 27-year-old man from Morocco who lives in Switzerland. He presents himself to the general practitioner, who has known him for a couple of years. He has experienced a good health, except for flu 2 years ago. Even though the patient's immigration is recent, his mastery of language and pronunciation are quite good. About 6 months ago the patient stayed 1 night on the department of neurology for the evaluation of the effects of a head trauma as result of an accident: quite unexpectedly, while riding a bicycle, he had been struck by a car. In addition to the commotio cerebri, he had a broken wrist, which recovered without functional restrictions. Four weeks after the accident, a neurologist saw the patient. His main complaints were difficulties with his capacity to concentrate and memorize.

The neurologist informed the general practitioner that the electroencephalograph did not show irregularities, and the neuropsychologic investigation also was normal except for unspecific and usual problems with concentration after a light head injury. The patient informed the general practitioner that ever since the accident there had been something wrong in his head. Although he has tried to explain this to the neurologist, the neurologist did not provide a clear answer, as far as the patient understood. The patient believes that the neurologist considered that his complaints were caused by nervousness. He is not satisfied, because his complaints do cause him concern. Because the patient presented the problem as an emergency and because the problem seemed complex, the patient was requested to return in the afternoon for a more intensive evaluation.

Additional information

In the afternoon the patient presented himself with his wife. He reports having frequent headaches and being tired without any effort; as a result, he does not feel he is able to work. In addition he has problems with his memory and is easily irritated. After the accident he tried once to return to his job, but this attempt failed because of the headaches. As a result he had a dispute with his company's medical officer. The patient informs the general practitioner that he is quite concerned about his health and that his health concerns preoccupy him most of the day. During the last month he has not slept well, and he feels tense, although he is not anxious. In addition, the patient recently lost some weight. As a Muslim, he does not smoke or drink alcohol. Compared with earlier visits, the general practitioner gets a different impression of the patient. The patient's mood seems low, and he is tense. The presentation of his story is clear and not confused. Physical examination, including the neurologic examination, does not provide evidence of a physical illness.

His wife provides the following information: She met him while on holiday in Morocco. She works in a flower shop and is in good physical health. According to his wife, their relationship has been increasingly tense in the last month. She has known him as an optimistic man who seemed to be quite capable of handling the problems of the last years. They had some friends who they saw on a regular basis, and they were considering having children. Although some friends had warned her about the problems of marrying a foreigner from such a different culture, she had been impressed with how he had adjusted to his new situation. There has been quite a change since the accident, however. The patient stays at home almost all day and does not do much, although cooking and reading always had his interest. He had become increasingly difficult and irritable. As a result, rather unexpectedly, their relationship had become difficult. After a quarrel last week over something unremarkable, she stayed for a night with her parents.

The patient was born in Casablanca. He comes from a stable family. He has two brothers who live in Europe. His parents died about a year ago, his mother after a short period of illness probably caused by a brain tumor, and his father as a result of a car accident. In Europe he has not been able to reach his former professional level as an electronic technician. At the time of the accident he was working as supervisor of a crew in a cleaning company. Recently, an employee has been fired for making discriminatory remarks to foreign colleagues, including the patient.

Scoring case 3

The reader is invited to score this case using scoring sheet provided in Fig. 8 and the clinical anchor points described in Appendix 1 and to check the results as presented at the end of Appendix 3.

	P	C	P
B	0 1 2 3 0 1 2 3	0 1 2 3 0 1 2 3	0 1 2 3
P	0 1 2 3 0 1 2 3	0 1 2 3 0 1 2 3	0 1 2 3
S	0 1 2 3 0 1 2 3	0 1 2 3 0 1 2 3	0 1 2 3
HC	0 1 2 3 0 1 2 3	0 1 2 3 0 1 2 3	0 1 2 3

Fig. 8. Scoring sheet for Case 3.

Case vignette

The patient is a 27-year-old Moroccan man, who sees his general practitioner for headaches and related physical problems that do not allow him to function as he is accustomed to doing. He is concerned. The symptoms have persisted since a commotio cerebri caused when a car hit his bicycle about 6 months ago. Recently he has been seen by a neurologist, who could not find a specific cause other than the accident. The patient has a stable living situation with his wife and is working as supervisor of a cleaning crew, although he is trained as an electronic technician. Recently he was the target of discrimination by a colleague at work because of his Muslim background.

He is a man who was able to enjoy himself. He and his wife always got along quite well, but recently they have had some quarrels related to his current state. He has always been able to handle problems in his life well. He neither drinks nor smokes. He has never had periods of psychologic dysfunctioning, except during the last month. He feels increasingly irritated and tense, and he cannot sleep. At the moment, nothing provides him much pleasure. Besides the hospital admission for the accident, the patient did not have any contacts with health care providers except for his general practitioner and the recent follow-up with the neurologist. This contact did not satisfy the patient; he felt he was not respected. The patient states that he is willing to do what the doctor suggests.

Treatment plan

Biologic. There is no evidence for a physical disease. There is need to monitor the patient's physical symptoms, but there is no need for further investigation.

Psychologic. There are no signs of previous vulnerability or poor coping. Because there is no history of somatization and poor coping, it is expected that a psychiatric diagnosis, including a clear explanation of the reason of his current state and his related concerns, will be an important first step in the treatment of the patient. It will provide a frame of reference for

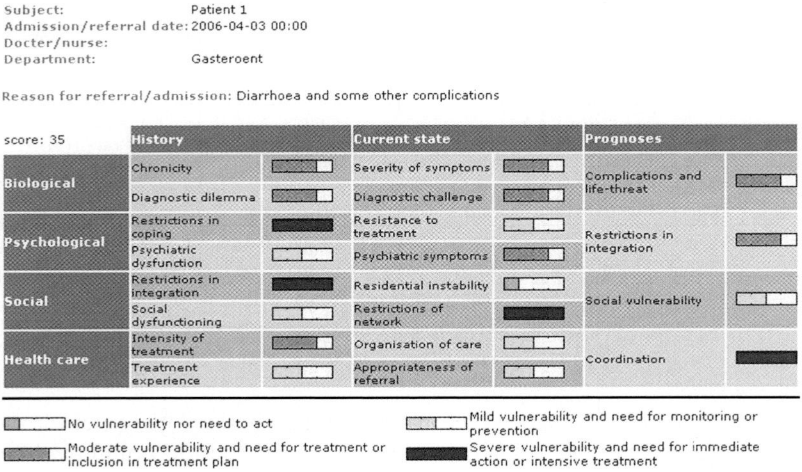

Subject: Patient 1
Admission/referral date: 2006-04-03 00:00
Docter/nurse:
Department: Gasteroent

Reason for referral/admission: Diarrhoea and some other complications

Fig. 9. Scoring of the case of patient 1.

treatment. In addition a psychologic intervention focusing on his hypochondriacal concerns, depressive cognitions, and his negative self-esteem intensified by the neglect he perceived during his interactions with the neurologist and his company's medical officer should reduce the patient's concerns and negative emotional state. Depending on the severity of depressive symptoms, antidepressants should be considered. His wife should be involved

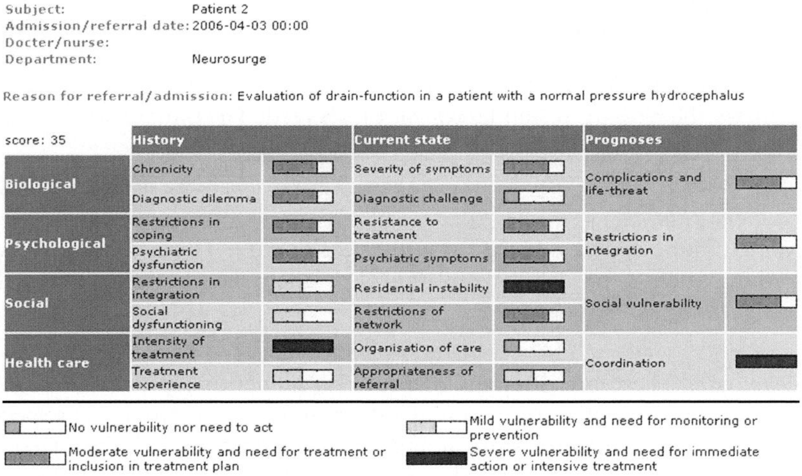

Subject: Patient 2
Admission/referral date: 2006-04-03 00:00
Docter/nurse:
Department: Neurosurge

Reason for referral/admission: Evaluation of drain-function in a patient with a normal pressure hydrocephalus

Fig. 10. Scoring of the case of patient 2.

Subject: Patient 3
Admission/referral date: 2006-04-03 00:00
Docter/nurse:
Department: General pr

Reason for referral/admission: Headache after an incident

score: 17

	History		Current state		Prognoses	
Biological	Chronicity		Severity of symptoms		Complications and life-threat	
	Diagnostic dilemma		Diagnostic challenge			
Psychological	Restrictions in coping		Resistance to treatment		Restrictions in integration	
	Psychiatric dysfunction		Psychiatric symptoms			
Social	Restrictions in integration		Residential instability		Social vulnerability	
	Social dysfunctioning		Restrictions of network			
Health care	Intensity of treatment		Organisation of care		Coordination	
	Treatment experience		Appropriateness of referral			

☐ No vulnerability nor need to act
☐ Mild vulnerability and need for monitoring or prevention
☐ Moderate vulnerability and need for treatment or inclusion in treatment plan
■ Severe vulnerability and need for immediate action or intensive treatment

Fig. 11. Scoring of the case of patient 3.

in the treatment, and the recent conflict resulting from the depression should be included as a focus of treatment.

Social. A plan for professional rehabilitation should be made.

Organization of care. This patient's case is not highly complex, as reflected in a total score of 17. Depending on his or her skills, the general practitioner should consider doing the assessment and the treatment as described. Alternately, the patient should be referred to a psychiatrist. Active coordination of care between the general practitioner and the company's medical officer (and the psychiatrist) is required. In this case, the coordination of care is primarily an exchange of diagnostic results and implementation of a subsequent integrated strategy.

Scoring of case examples

Figs. 9, 10, and 11 show the scoring of patients 1, 2, and 3, respectively.

References

[1] Ormel J, VonKorff M, Ustun TB, et al. Common mental disorders and disability across cultures: results from the WHO collaborative study on psychological problems in general health care. JAMA 1994;272:1471–8.
[2] De Groot M, Anderson R, Freedland KE, et al. Association of depression and diabetes complications: a meta analysis. Psychosom Med 2001;63:619–30.
[3] Ciechanowski PS, Katon WJ, Russo JE. Depression and diabetes: impact of depressive symptoms on adherence, function and costs. Arch Intern Med 2000;160:3278–85.

[4] De Jonge P, Ormel J, Slaets JPJ, et al. Depressive symptoms in the elderly predict poor adjustment following somatic events. Am J Geriatr Psychiatry 2004;12:57–64.

[5] Wulsin LR, Vaillant GE, Wells VE. A systematic review of the mortality of depression. Psychosom Med 1999;61(1):6–17.

[6] Dimatteo MR, Lepper HS, Croghan TW. Depression is a risk factor for noncompliance with medical treatment. Arch Intern Med 2000;160:2101–7.

[7] de Jonge P, Ormel J, van den Brink RHS, et al. Symptom dimensions of depression following myocardial infarction and their relationship with somatic health status and cardiovascular prognosis. Am J Psychiatry 2006;163(1):138–44.

[8] Engel GL. The need for a new medical model: a challenge for biomedicine. Science 1977;196: 129–36.

[9] Kessler D, Lloyd K, Lewis G, et al. Cross sectional study of symptom attribution and recognition of depression and anxiety in primary care. BMJ 1999;318:436–9.

[10] Penn JV, Boland R, McCartney JR, et al. Recognition and treatment of depressive disorders by internal medicine attendings and housestaff. Gen Hosp Psychiatry 1997;19:179–84.

[11] Leigh H, Feinstein AR, Reiser MF. The patient evaluation grid: a systematic approach to comprehensive care. Gen Hosp Psychiatry 1980;2:3–9.

[12] Huyse FJ. From consult to complexity of care prediction and health services needs assessment. J Psychosom Res 1997;43:233–40.

[13] Huyse FJ, Lyons JS, Stiefel FC, et al. "INTERMED": a method to assess health service needs: I. development and first results on its reliability. Gen Hosp Psychiatry 1999;21: 39–48.

[14] Stiefel FC, de Jonge P, Huyse FJ, et al. "INTERMED": a method to assess health service needs: II. Results on its validity and clinical use. Gen Hosp Psychiatry 1999;21:49–56.

[15] Huyse FJ, Lyons JS, Stiefel FC, et al. Operationalizing the biopsychosocial model. The INTERMED [editorial]. Psychosomatics 2001;42–1:5–13.

[16] Boenink AD, Huyse FJ. Arie Querido (1901–1983), a Dutch psychiatrist. His views on integrated health care. J Psychosom Res 1997;43:551–7.

[17] Nurcombe B, Gallagher RM. The clinical process in psychiatry. Cambridge: Cambridge University Press; 1986.

[18] Lyons JS, Howard KI, O'Mahoney MT, et al. The measurement and management of clinical outcomes in mental health. New York: John Wisely & Sons; 1997.

[19] Huyse FJ, Herzog T, Malt UF, et al. A screening instrument for the detection of psychosocial risk factors in patients admitted to general hospital wards, (grantnumber: BMH1–CT93–1180). In: Baert EA, editor. Biomedical and health research. The BIOMED1 programme. Bruxelles, Belgium: Ohmsha IOS Press; 1995. p. 496–7.

[20] Huyse FJ, de Jonge P, Slaets JP, et al. COMPRI—an instrument to detect patients with complex care needs: results from a European study. Psychosomatics 2001;42(3):222–8.

[21] Fink P. Mental illness and admission to general hospitals: a register investigation. Acta Psychiatr Scand 1990;82:458–62.

[22] Covinsky KE, Fortinsky RH, Palmer RM, et al. Relation between symptoms of depression and health status outcomes in acutely ill hospitalized older persons. Ann Intern Med 1997; 126:417–25.

[23] Beitman BD, Mukerji V, Lamberti JW, et al. Panic disorder in patients with chest pain and angiographically normal coronary arteries. Am J Cardiol 1989;63:1399–403.

[24] Jones PW, Baveystock CM, Littlejohns P. Relationships between general health measured with the sickness impact profile and respiratory symptoms, physiological measures, and mood in patients with chronic airflow limitation. Am Rev Respir Dis 1989;140(6): 1538–43.

[25] Saravay SM, Lavin M. Psychiatric comorbidity and length of stay in the general hospital. A critical review of outcome studies. Psychosomatics 1995;3:233–52.

[26] Browne GB, Arpin K, Corey P, et al. Individual correlates of health service utilisation and the cost of poor adjustment to chronic illness. Med Care 1990;28:43–58.

[27] Katon W, VonKorff M, Lin E, et al. Distressed high utilizers of medical care. DSM-III-R diagnoses and treatment needs. Gen Hosp Psychiatry 1990;12:355–62.

[28] Berkman B, Walker S, Bonander E, et al. Early unplanned readmissions to social work of elderly patients: factors predicting who needs follow-up services. Soc Work Health Care 1992;17:103–19.

[29] Johnson J, Weissman MM, Klerman GL. Service utilization and social morbidity associated with depressive symptoms in the community. JAMA 1992;267:1478–83.

[30] Kessler LG, Burns BJ, Shapiro S, et al. Psychiatric diagnoses of medical service users: evidence from the Epidemiologic Catchment Area Program. Am J Public Health 1987;77: 18–24.

[31] Horn SD. Validity, reliability and implications of an index of patient severity of illness. Med Care 1981;19:354–9.

[32] Haynes RB, Taylor DW, Sackett DL. Compliance in health care. Baltimore (MD): Johns Hopkins University Press; 1979.

[33] Institute of Medicine. Crossing the quality chasm: a new health system for the 21st century. Committee on Quality of Health Care in America. Washington (DC): National Academy Press; 2001.

[34] Gordon M. Nursing diagnosis: process and application. 3rd edition. Philadelphia: Elsevier; 1994.

[35] Nunnally J. Psychometric theory. New York: John Wiley & Sons; 1976.

[36] Feinstein AR. Multi-item "instruments" vs Virginia Apgar's principles of clinimetrics. Arch Intern Med 1999;159:125–8.

[37] Endicott J, Spitzer RL, Fleiss JL, et al. The global assessment scale. A procedure for measuring overall severity of psychiatric disturbance. Arch Gen Psychiatry 1976;33(6):766–71.

[38] Crocker L, Algina J. Introduction to classical and modern test theory. New York: Holt, Rinehart and Winston; 1991.

[39] De Jonge P, Ruinemans GMF, Huyse FJ, et al. A simple risk score predicts poor quality of life and non-survival at one year follow up in dialysis patients. Nephrol Dial Transplant 2003;18:2622–8.

[40] De Jonge P, Latour C, Huyse FJ. Inter-rater reliability of the INTERMED in a heterogeneous somatic population. J Psychosom Res 2002;52:25–7.

[41] De Jonge P, Hoogervorst ELJ, Huyse FJ, et al. INTERMED: temporal stability in a sample of MS patients. Gen Hosp Psychiatry 2004;6:147–52.

[42] De Jonge P, Stiefel FC. Internal consistency of the INTERMED in patients with somatic diseases. J Psychosom Res 2002;54:497–9.

[43] De Jonge P, Huyse FJ, Stiefel FC, et al. INTERMED—a clinical instrument for biopsychosocial assessment. Psychosomatics 2001;42:106–9.

[44] De Jonge P, Bauer I, Huyse FJ, et al. Medical inpatients at risk of extended hospital stay and poor discharge health status: detection with COMPRI and INTERMED. Psychosom Med 2003;65:534–41.

[45] Fischer CJ, Stiefel FC, de Jonge P, et al. Case complexity and clinical outcome in diabetes mellitus: a prospective study using the INTERMED. Diabetes Metab 2000;26:295–302.

[46] Hoogervorst ELJ, de Jonge P, Huyse FJ, et al. The INTERMED: a screening instrument to identify multiple sclerosis patients in need of multi-disciplinary treatment. J Neurol Neurosurg Psychiatry 2003;74:20–4.

[47] Koch N, Stiefel F, de Jonge P, et al. Identification of case complexity and increased health care utilization in patients with rheumatoid arthritis. Arthritis Rheum 2001;45(3):216–21.

[48] de Jonge P, Huyse FJ, Slaets JP, et al. Operationalization of biopsychosocial case complexity in general health care: the INTERMED project. Aust N Z J Psychiatry 2005;39(9):795–9.

[49] Ludwig G, Michaud L, Berney S, et al. The biopsychosocial screening of transplant patients by means of the INTERMED. J Psychosom Res 2005;59:38.

[50] Stiefel F, Bel Hadj B, Zdrojewski C, et al. A randomised psychiatric intervention in complex medical patients: effects on depression. J Psychosom Res 2004;56:578–9.

[51] De Jonge P, Latour C, Huyse FJ. Implementing psychiatric interventions on a general medical ward: effects on patients' quality of life and length of hospital stay. Psychosom Med
2003;65:997–1002.
[52] Kathol RG, McAlpine D, Kishi Y, et al. General medical and pharmacy claims expenditures
in users of behavioral health services. J Gen Intern Med 2005;20(2):160–7.

ELSEVIER
SAUNDERS

THE MEDICAL
CLINICS
OF NORTH AMERICA

Med Clin N Am 90 (2006) 759–760

Reflections and Perspectives

Friedrich C. Stiefel, MD, PhD[a],*,
Frits J. Huyse, MD, PhD[b]

[a]*Service de Psychiatrie de Liaison, Centre Hospitalier Universitaire Vaudois,
Rue du Bugnon 44, CH-1011 Lausanne, Switzerland*
[b]*Department of General Internal Medicine, University Medical Center Groningen,
Hanzeplein 1, 9700 RB, Groningen, The Netherlands*

Although systems can be broken down into parts that are interesting in and of themselves, the real power lies in the way that the parts come together and are interconnected to fulfil some purpose [1]. This statement is certainly true for the complex patient who encounters a complex medical system [2,3].

As soon as interconnections can be identified (eg, the interdependencies between biologic, psychologic, and social factors of illnesses or the links between increased medical care use of patients for whom the medical system does not find any organic cause of their suffering) and the power of the underlying dynamics can be understood, a given situation often can be perceived as less chaotic or even meaningful and a controlled approach becomes possible.

Complex patients who have biopsychosocial comorbidities represent a major challenge for the current health care system. Unlike standard medical situations for which medical care can be based on an evidence-based approach, complex patients require a broader concept of care. As demonstrated throughout this issue, such an integrated approach that takes into account the concepts of case- and care complexity is not only possible, it is cost-effective. Integrated care, however, needs assessment tools and a communications-based approach that fosters exchange and collaboration between different medical disciplines and professions and patients.

Theoretic understanding, conceptual and operational frameworks, and scientific evidence are all necessary, yet are not sufficient conditions for the improvement in care of the complex patient. As with any other change,

* Corresponding author.
E-mail address: frederic.stiefel@chuv.ch (F.C. Stiefel).

0025-7125/06/$ - see front matter © 2006 Elsevier Inc. All rights reserved.
doi:10.1016/j.mcna.2006.04.004
medical.theclinics.com

a change in medical practice depends on strong incentives. Some of the most powerful incentives in the current health care system and in our society are economic savings and cost-effectiveness. The important medical progress of the last decades and the associated heavy burden of financial costs may be a key element of change. While medicine of the past had to face the limits of knowledge and skills, modern medicine will face limited financial resources that will restrict the therapeutic options. Before limiting access to medical treatments, medicine will be asked to enhance cost-effectiveness.

The complex medical patient is a source of important health care use with low cost-effectiveness. Therefore, integrated care of the complex medical patient represents a necessary and innovative alternative to current medical practice. To achieve such a change in the paradigm of care of the complex medical patient, 10 rules for reaching these goals were described in the preface (see elsewhere in this issue) [3]. These imply that different players in the health care system will have to realize the advantages of a change toward integrated care: the clinicians who work in primary care and in the general hospitals, the mental health care professionals, the patients, the policy makers and insurance companies, the hospital managers, and politicians. All of them, as well as the complex patient and the society as a whole would benefit from such a change.

References

[1] Plesk PE, Wilson T. Complexity, leadership, and management in healthcare organizations. BMJ 2001;323:746–9.
[2] Institute of Medicine. Crossing the quality chasm: a new health system for the 21st century. Committee on Quality of Health Care in America. Washington DC: National Academy Press; 2001.
[3] Wilson T, Holt T. Complexity and clinical care. BMJ 2001;323:685–8.

ELSEVIER
SAUNDERS

Med Clin N Am 90 (2006) 761–767

THE MEDICAL
CLINICS
OF NORTH AMERICA

Index

Note: Page numbers of article titles are in **boldface** type.

Moving?

Make sure your subscription moves with you!

To notify us of your new address, find your **Clinics Account Number** (located on your mailing label above your name), and contact customer service at:

E-mail: elspcs@elsevier.com

800-654-2452 (subscribers in the U.S. & Canada)
407-345-4000 (subscribers outside of the U.S. & Canada)

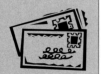

Fax number: 407-363-9661

Elsevier Periodicals Customer Service
6277 Sea Harbor Drive
Orlando, FL 32887-4800

*To ensure uninterrupted delivery of your subscription, please notify us at least 4 weeks in advance of move.